I Can't Believe It's Yoga
for Pregnancy and After!

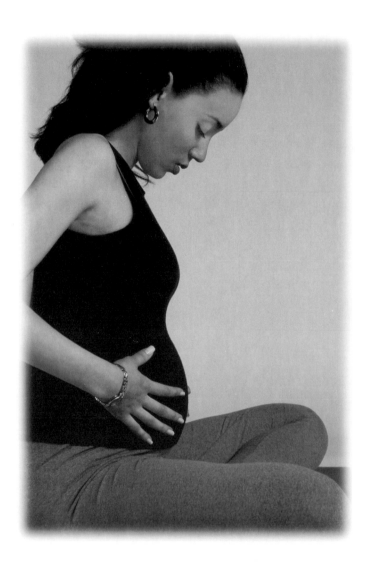

I Can't Believe It's Yoga for Pregnancy and After!

Lisa Trivell

Photos by Peter Field Peck

Hatherleigh Press
New York

A Getfitnow.com book

I Can't Believe It's Yoga for Pregnancy and After!
A Getfitnow.com Book

Hatherleigh Press/Getfitnow.com Books
An Affiliate of W.W. Norton & Company, Inc.
500 Fifth Ave
New York, NY 10110
1-800-528-2500

Visit our website: www.getfitnow.com

Disclaimer:

Before beginning any strenuous exercise program consult your physician. The
author and publisher of this book and workout disclaim any liability, personal or
professional, resulting from the misapplication of any of the training procedures
described in this publication.

All Getfitnow.com titles are available for bulk purchase, special
promotions, and premiums. For more information, please contact the manager
of our Special Sales Department at 1-800-528-2500.

Library of Congress Cataloging-in-Publication Data
Trivell, Lisa. 1956-
    I can't believe it's yoga for pregnancy and after/Lisa Trivell.
      p. cm.
    ISBN 1-57826-046-9 (alk.paper)
    1. Exercise for pregnant women. 2. Yoga, Hatha. 3. Prenatal care.
4.Postnatal care.
    RG558.7 .T75 2000
    618.2'4--dc21   00-031938

Cover design by Lisa Fyfe
Text design and composition by dcdesigns

Photographed by Peter Field Peck
with Canon® cameras and lenses on Fuji® slide film
Printed in Canada on acid-free paper
10 9 8 7 6 5 4 3 2 1

To my two children, Amanda and Dylan,
and to the children of the parents in this book.

ACKNOWLEDGEMENTS

There are a lot of people that have helped to create this book. I am so grateful to the mothers, fathers and child that have been studying yoga with me and are pictured in the book—Roxanne Hughes, Bridget LeRoy and Eric Johnson in the prenatal section, and Tonia, John and Cameron Kavanaugh, who modeled for the postnatal section. Thank you so much for participating in the book.

I'd like to thank my husband and two children, Amanda and Dylan.

Thanks to the team at Hatherleigh Press and Getfitnow.com for believing in this project and the two prior books in the *I Can't Believe It's Yoga* series.

Tracy Tumminello deserves a special thank-you for her expert editing and organizational skills.

My publisher Andrew Flach for his vision to put together the *I Can't Believe It's Yoga* series.

And Peter Field Peck, for his talented photography and enthusiasm.

PART I: INTRODUCTION

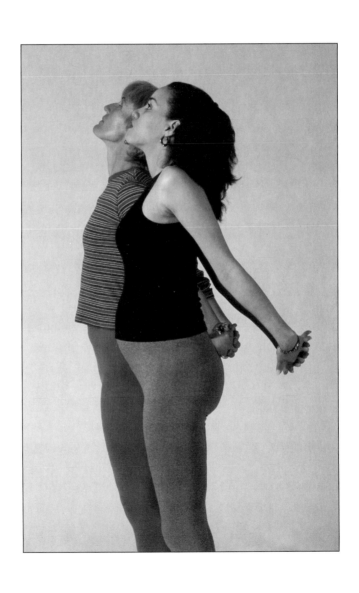

Today, more and more women are realizing the importance of continuing to exercise throughout their pregnancy. Yoga is a perfect form of exercise to practice during pregnancy because of its gentle yet effective nature, working the body from the inside out and incorporating important breathing techniques useful during labor. Pregnancy is an incredible time in your life. There's no need for you to feel uncomfortable and achy when you can take advantage of all the benefits of yoga and exercise.

You should enjoy your pregnancy; it is the time nature gives you to nurture your baby and prepare to become a parent. I have two children. I loved being pregnant and had relatively easy births. I believe that this was partly due to genetics and partly because I practiced and taught yoga throughout both pregnancies. I also treated myself to regular massages more often during this period of my life. The combination of doing yoga and receiving massage when you are pregnant brings numerous benefits. Both help alleviate many adverse effects and discomforts of pregnancy such as, muscular tension, headaches, tiredness, nausea, weakness, mood swings, and Sciatica.

No two pregnancies are exactly alike. You may experience emotional highs and lows, anticipation, fear, peacefulness and excitement. All of these emotions are normal.

Pregnancy is a very special time–exciting as well as a little scary. It is a time of transition; changing self-images; physical, mental, and spiritual growth; commitment; and miracles. It is a time when your consciousness and your baby are housed in one body.

Yoga will help you to cope with all the physical and hormonal changes that occur. During pregnancy your body opens in many ways–your rib cage expands to take in more oxygen; your pelvis becomes more flexible to enable the baby to pass through; your mind is open to new ideas and an increased inner awareness.

Each woman starts her pregnancy at a different stage of fitness. The amount and intensity of your workout will depend on your own fitness level. Some women might be aerobic training or taking yoga classes regularly at the start of their pregnancy, others may be used to doing some moderate exercise, while some may not exercise at all and see pregnancy as a time to start. Women not accustomed to exercising should proceed carefully into an exercise program.

In addition to yoga, massage can help relax both the mother and baby before and after birth. Practicing massage techniques with your partner is a wonderful way to interact in a sensual and intimate way during pregnancy, as well as a nurturing and exciting way to interact with your baby after delivery.

The massage techniques and yoga positions presented in this book are for the beginner and more experienced yoga enthusiasts alike. Adapt these routines to your workout before pregnancy and continue them after your baby arrives.

–Lisa Trivell

PART II: WHY DO YOGA?

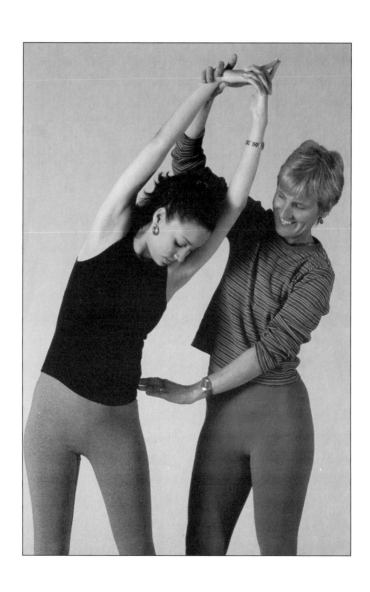

Yoga integrates the body and mind through concentrating on the breath. Of course being aware of your breathing and knowing many different breathing techniques will be very helpful throughout your pregnancy, as well as during your baby's birth and postnatal. In addition, yoga helps you feel more balanced in body, mind and emotion.

Yoga enables you to get a well-rounded workout, which tones and stretches many muscle groups. You will exercise muscles you know you have, in addition to muscles, tendons and ligaments of which you are not even aware!

BENEFITS OF YOGA

1. Maintains or improves maternal fitness and posture
2. Improves mental outlook and self-image
3. Increases energy
4. Improves sleep
5. Balances hormones
6. Reduces backaches
7. Reduces water retention
8. Improves circulation
9. Reduces leg cramps
10. Reduces Varicose veins
11. Decreases anxiety, boosts your emotional state
12. Prevents headaches
13. Eases gastrointestinal discomforts, such as heartburn and constipation
14. Increases stamina, aiding pain endurance during labor
15. Strengthens birthing muscles
16. Quickens postpartum recovery
17. Reduces need for medical interventions (e.g. pitocen use, forceps delivery, cesarean section)
18. Increases chance of natural birth
19. Shortens pushing stage
20. Facilitates getting back into shape after birth
21. Reduces stretch marks by distributing weight gain more evenly and gradually

The Research

Here's what some research says about the value of yoga and exercise during pregnancy:

A study by the American College of Obstetrics and Gynecologists looked at pregnant women who participated in fitness programs. The active women reported that exercise decreased the discomforts of pregnancy, relieved tension and improved self image.

A study published in the *Journal of Medicine and Science in Sports* and Exercise found that women who

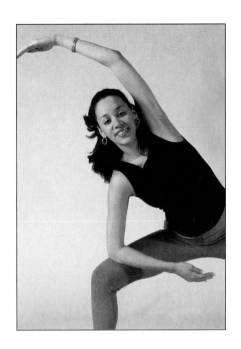

continued to exercise three times a week for 30 minutes each session, gained less weight overall and put on less body fat than women who quit exercising during pregnancy. In addition, researchers at Ohio College of Medicine found that women who participated in prenatal fitness exercises, experienced shorter pushing stages during labor. Labor may be shorter due to increased strength and flexibility, and a greater awareness of using the breathing techniques and pelvic floor muscles.

Other research suggests women who practice yoga are less likely to suffer common pregnancy discomforts such as swelling and nausea. When I was pregnant, I would encourage myself to do yoga even when I felt nauseous, and I would always feel better.

Yoga is a gentle workout, especially beneficial to women during the childbearing months. Its exercises are safe and will help you feel great. Yoga will not overheat your body. It will help you feel physically and psychologically healthy, especially if you start practicing yoga before your pregnancy. *A woman who feels strong and in control of her body before pregnancy, will be more likely to feel secure and less anxious during labor and delivery.*

7

PART III: PREGNANCY AND YOUR BODY

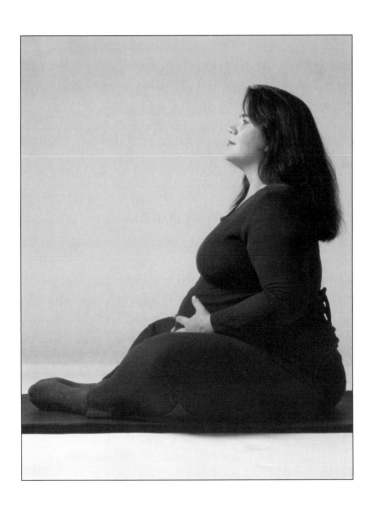

During pregnancy your body performs like a highly efficient factory. Every system of your body changes. Some symptoms of these changes are visible while others are not. Although pregnancy is a highly individual experience, many of the physical and psychological changes are similar. A discussion of the most common changes and how yoga can help follows.

Metabolic Changes

One change is an altered metabolism. During pregnancy your body has to get nutrition to the fetus, resulting in a necessary total weight gain of 24 to 30 pounds (averaging 2.5 lbs. the first trimester, 10 lbs. the second trimester, and 11 lbs. the third trimester).

Because of this weight gain, you need to strengthen the muscles in your back and shoulders to make it easier to stand and sit up straight. Strengthening your back through yoga also will be beneficial when it comes time to nurse and carry your child. During the later stages of pregnancy, you will especially appreciate yoga and massage because your lower back can get so tired.

Changes in Oxygen Demand

The amount of oxygen your body needs increases as your pregnancy progresses, with your body requiring one third more oxygen just to do light exercise. This is all due to the increased demands of the fetus, placenta and uterus. Yoga teaches you to breathe fully so that even as your stomach grows, you learn to expand your ribcage and fully engage your lungs.

Cardiovascular Changes

Pregnancy requires 50 percent more work from the heart. The increase peaks at the seventh month and holds steady through delivery. During labor the heart has to work even harder. Blood volume increases by 40 percent, and resting heart rate increases by 10 to 15 beats a minute. You can sometimes feel tired or get easily out of breath if you have not been exercising before your pregnancy. A woman who maintains fitness during pregnancy can meet the demands of carrying and delivering her baby.

The cardiovascular system pumps blood throughout the entire body. Dramatic changes occur in this system during pregnancy. Arteries tend to dilate, resulting in lower blood pressure. This can lead to temporary weakness and dizziness during strenuous exercise. Yoga is not strenuous as long as you increase length and demand slowly. Always be sure to bring your head up last to reduce light-headedness.

Muscular and Anatomical Changes

Pregnancy affects your muscles in many ways. Increased levels of the hormones estrogen and relaxin cause elasticity of the joints, ligaments and connective tissue, posing an increased risk of injury. It is very important to strengthen the muscle groups that support the joints. Increased hormone levels can also cause changes in skin complexion. Yoga will reduce the risk of injury, as well as increase circulation, which helps to control hormones.

The necessary weight you are gaining during your pregnancy causes an imbalance in your body. To avoid spasms and knots developing in your muscles and to maintain good posture during pregnancy, it is important to balance the muscles on both sides of your body through yoga. Increased breast size can also affect posture. Through yoga, you expand your chest and strengthen your back. Balancing poses are included in this book and are very important to incorporate into your routine. They help you to center your mind and body.

Energy expenditure increases as pregnancy advances. When you hold tension in your body and mind, you get tired. Yoga increases circulation and helps to relieve stress so you have more energy. It also helps to increase red blood cell count, which lessens fatigue.

Since there is an increase in the size and shape of the uterus, it is recommended that you do not lie on your back for more then a few minutes at a time after 20 weeks of pregnancy. Whenever possible, lie on your left side.

Respiratory Changes

Breathlessness and hyperventilation are common in later pregnancy, because the enlarging uterus compresses the diaphragm. Yoga can relieve this by stretching the torso and encouraging full use of the lungs.

Set a goal to do yoga everyday. Some days you may practice for 15 minutes; other days for 20 minutes or a half hour. You also should take an hour once a week to work with your partner doing double yoga, massage and guided relaxation. The key is to pace yourself and do some yoga daily. On page 171, you will find yoga workouts to fit a variety of time frames.

Remember, yoga is not strenuous as long as you increase length and demand gradually. In the later stages of your pregnancy, it is important not to drop your head below your knees. Always roll your back up slowly, bringing your head up last.

PART IV: PRENATAL EXERCISES

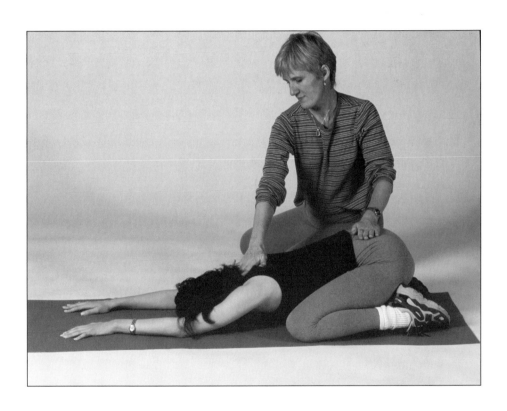

Many of the exercises in this book can be done throughout your pregnancy. If, however, any of them become uncomfortable or straining, they should be reduced or eliminated. It is also important to take brisk walks or swim during your pregnancy for some gentle aerobic exercise. During the last six weeks of your pregnancy, when you may experience lower back fatigue, breathlessness, and lightheadedness, you may want to do the modified workout, listed in the workout section.

Remember:

1. Check with your doctor before beginning any exercise program.
2. Be careful not to over-stretch the Diatasis Rectus (the ligament running down the center of your stomach.) Intense abdominal exercise can separate this fragile ligament, especially in the third trimester.
3. Be consistent. Do some exercise everyday.
4. Wear loose, comfortable clothes.
5. Try to practice yoga on a yoga mat.
6. Be sure to practice in a room with good ventilation and at a comfortable temperature.
7. Soft music is recommended to help you relax and remain focused.
8. Always go to your personal degree of stretch or strength. Stretch until you feel discomfort, take a breath, and then try stretching a little further.
9. Do not continue the exercise if you feel pain. Stop and rest, or try a different exercise.
10. Always incorporate your breathing. Remember to exhale as much as you inhale.
11. Take time in between the exercises to be aware your breathing.
12. Do not worry about when to inhale and exhale–just don't hold your breath. Integration of your breath will come naturally as you practice.

Breathing Exercises

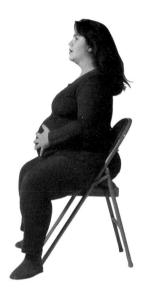 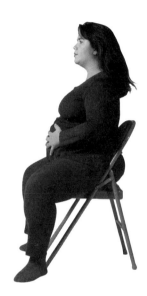

Rock-the-Baby Breath—This exercise can be done on a mat or in a chair. Cross your legs. Place your hands over your stomach and focus on the baby growing inside you. Breathe through your nose unless you are congested. Feel your belly rock forward as you inhale and feel it rock back to your spine as you exhale. As you progress in your pregnancy, imagine rocking your baby gently forward and back in your belly.

Benefit: tones the internal stomach muscles, prepares the mother for birth, soothes the baby growing inside and relaxes the mother.

Three Part Breath—Involves using the abdominal or baby area while taking deep breaths and concentrating on each breath. Your stomach will expand as you inhale, and contract as you exhale. In order to take deep breaths you have to learn to relax your abdominal muscles. When this breath is first explained, many people find that they do just the opposite. It is much easier to learn this breath when you are pregnant because your stomach is prominent. Inhale. Count to four and feel your lungs expand towards the back, sides and front. Hold for two counts. Exhale and empty your lungs to the count of four. This breathing routine is great for the last month of pregnancy.

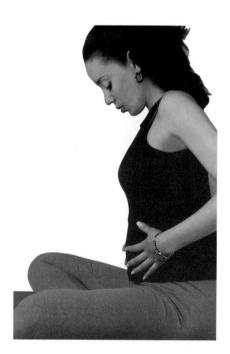

Benefit: encourages deep full breath using full lung capacity, expands the ribcage and the muscles between the ribs, teaches breath control.

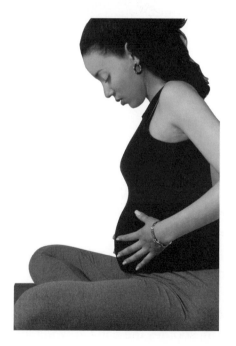

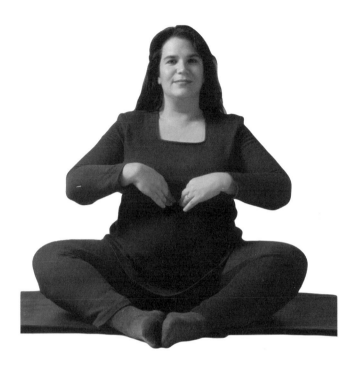

Bunny Breath—Relax your abdominal muscles completely in order to do this exercise effectively. Take short breaths, inhaling through the nose exhaling through the mouth or the nose. On each exhale, contract your abdominals. Breathe slowly ten times and then more quickly, ten times. Concentrate on your lower abdominals.

Benefit: helps prepare for labor, invigorates breath if you are feeling sluggish, and tones the abdominal muscles.

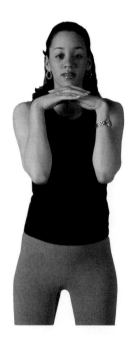
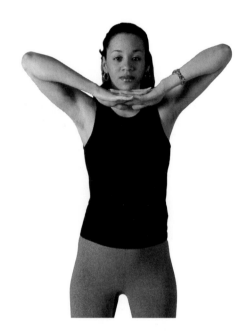

Angel Breath—Stand in mountain pose (described on page 32) and interlace your fingers under your chin. Inhale as you lift your elbows up. Exhale and drop them back down. Breathe through your nose, inhaling and exhaling completely.

Benefit: helps to fill the lungs especially in later pregnancy or when having heartburn. Also uses the intercostal muscles, in between the ribs, which can get tight.

SEATED EXERCISES

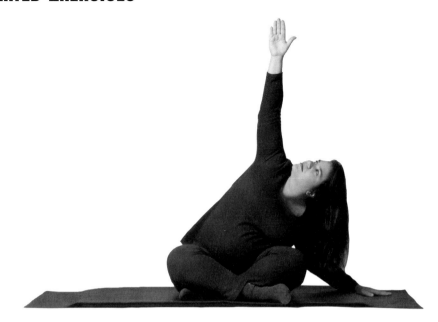

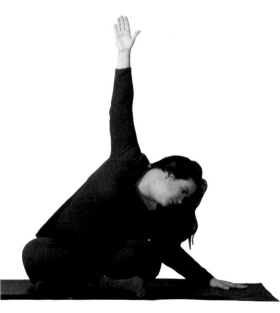

Seated Side Stretch—Sit cross-legged, hips planted. Stretch over to your left side by stretching your right arm up to the sky or over your ear. Breathe fully and then stretch over to the right. Breathe. Repeat three times.

Benefit: tones the hips and waist, releases tension in the shoulders.

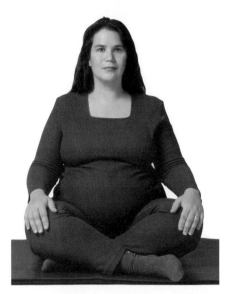 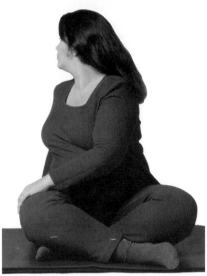

Cross-Legged Spinal Twist—Sit cross-legged with your right hand on your left knee and your left hand on the ground close to your lower back. Inhale as you lengthen your spine. Exhale and gently twist, from your tailbone up through your neck. Repeat twice. Then twist in the other direction.

Benefit: helps to balance the nervous system, releases tension along the spine.

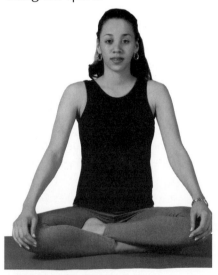 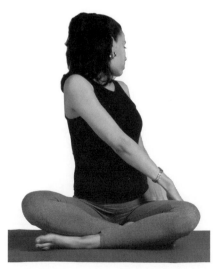

Chin Rolls—Sit cross-legged comfortably, with your hands on your knees. Drop your right ear toward your right shoulder and inhale. Bring your chin down to your chest and exhale. Then, move your left ear toward your left shoulder and inhale. Keep your shoulders down and your chest open. Repeat three times.

Benefit: relaxes and tones sides and back of your neck.

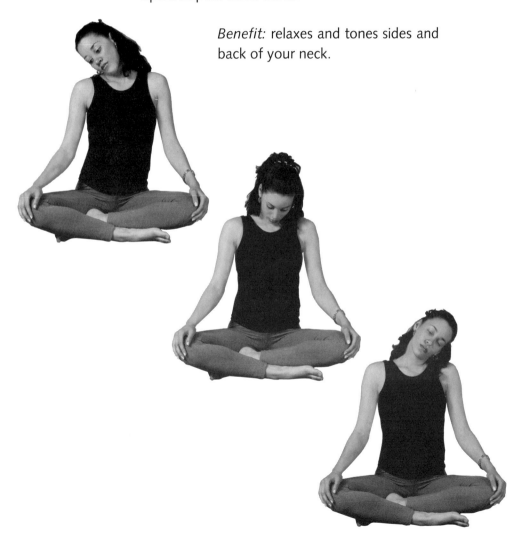

Neck Stretch—Sit cross-legged (you may prop a small pillow under your hips for additional comfort). Make sure you are already warmed up. Drop your left ear toward your left shoulder. Press your left hand over your right ear, and take two full breaths. Slowly reverse to the other side.

Benefit: very effective stretch for the side of your neck.

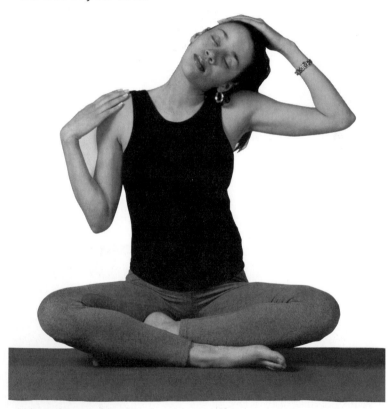

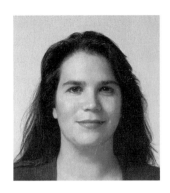

Eye Exercises—Sit cross-legged, drop your shoulders, lift your chest and lengthen your neck. Without moving your head, look all the way up with your eyes, look as far as you can to the right, all the way down, then all the way to the left. Make three complete circles to the right. Rest, and then perform three complete circles to the left. Rest.

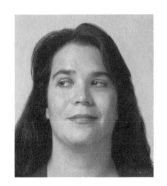

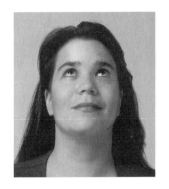

Benefit: relieves tired eyes and headaches.

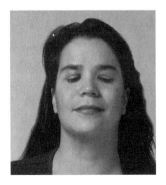

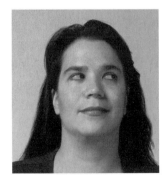

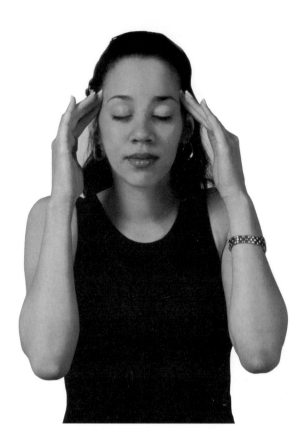

Temple Self-Massage—Sit cross-legged (you may prop a small pillow under your hips for additional comfort). With the index finger and middle finger of both hands gently touch your scalp and make small circles around the temples. Repeat three times in each direction.

Benefit: relieves headaches and scalp tension.

Butterfly—Sit on your sit bones with knees apart, feet together. Inhale as you lengthen your spine and drop your shoulders. (As you progress in your pregnancy you will find it is more comfortable to move the feet farther out in front of you.) Bend your elbows, dropping your chin towards your feet on the exhale. Repeat three times.

Benefit: Increases strength and flexibility in the hips, releases tightness in the lower back.

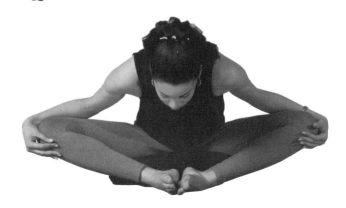

Butterfly Foot Massage—Sit in the butterfly pose with your pinky toes together and your big toes apart. Using your thumbs, make small circular strokes from your heels to the balls of your feet. Be sensitive to tightness and repeat stroking where it is tight.

Benefit: increases circulation in the feet, helps the back through reflexology.

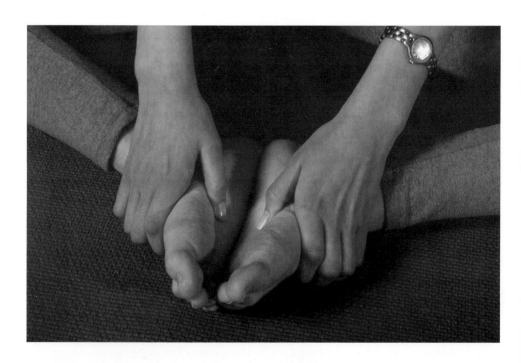

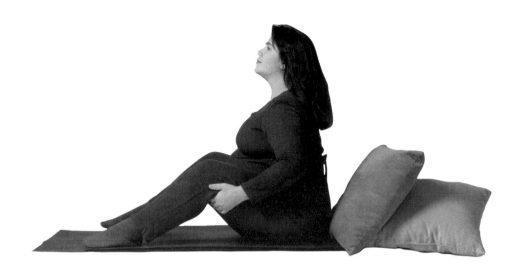

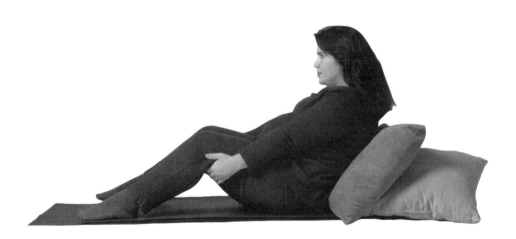

Roll Backs—Place a big pillow behind you. Sit with your knees bent, hands placed under your thighs. As you exhale, tilt your pelvis and round your back slightly, feeling your abdominals engage. Inhale and tilt your torso back up. Repeat three to eight times.

Benefit: tones lower abdominals while protecting the stomach muscles from over stretching.

27

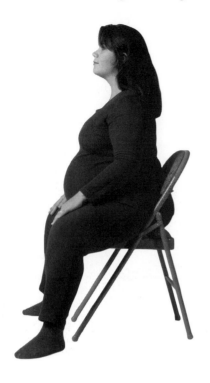

Seated Roll Down—Sit on a chair with your legs comfortably apart. Roll down head—first one vertebra at a time, relaxing your back as you roll. (Do not drop your head below the knees if you are in the third trimester.) Slowly roll back up head last.

Benefit: relaxes your entire back and your hips.

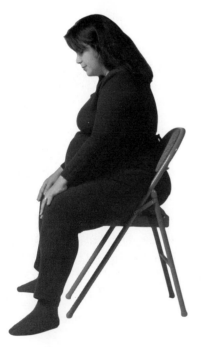

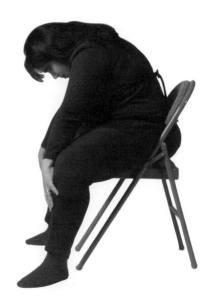

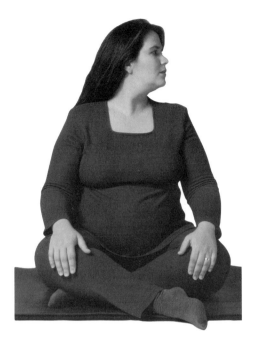

Side to Side Neck Stretch—Sit in a comfortable cross-legged position, hands on your knees. Turn your head all the way to the right, chin stretching toward your shoulder. Breathe fully. Move your head through the middle then stretch over your left shoulder. Breathe. Return to center. Repeat.

Benefit: exercises the sides of the neck, improves posture.

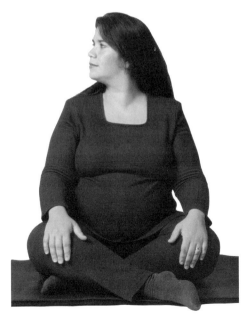

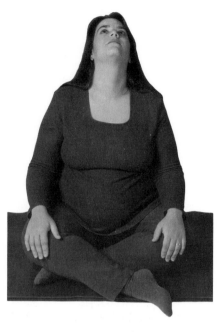 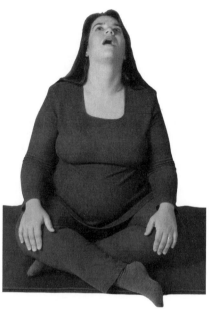

Mouth Exercise—Tilt your head back and open your jaw. Scoop your bottom row of teeth down and in front of your top teeth.

Benefit: releases tightness in the jaw, tones the neck muscles. It is important not to tighten your jaw during labor.

STANDING EXERCISES

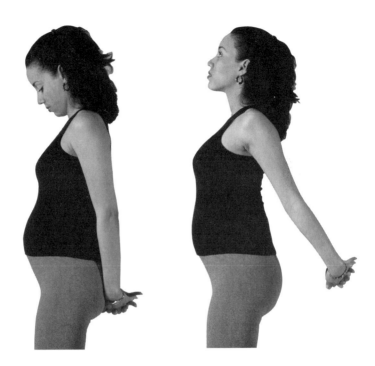

Chest Expansion—Stand with your legs hips-width apart, arms interlaced behind you and your chin down. As you inhale, expand your chest raising your arms and chin. Repeat three times.

Benefit: improves posture especially rounded shoulders, releases tension between the ribs and around the shoulder blades.

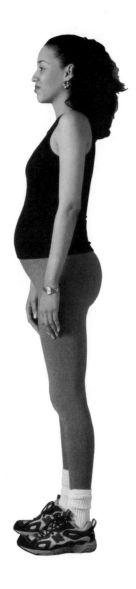

Mountain Pose—Stand with your feet parallel and hips-width apart. Lengthen your spine, drop your shoulders, and make sure that your chin is parallel to the ground.

Benefit: Good starter position for other poses, and is a great exercise for posture awareness.

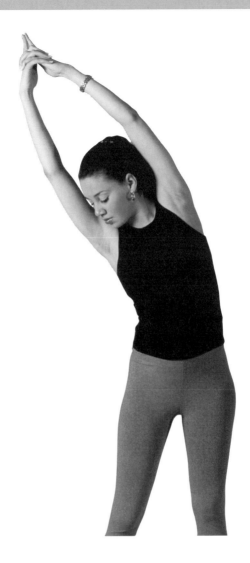

Half Moon—Stand with your feet hips-width apart, interlace your fingers overhead and stretch your arms to the right, hips to the left. Hold the position and take a full breath. Change sides. Repeat three times on each side.

Benefit: releases tension in the shoulders, tones the waist, and encourages full breathing.

Forward Bend—Stand with your feet parallel, knees bent and slowly roll down your back vertebra by vertebra. Then, roll up vertebra by vertebra lifting your head last.

Benefit: great for releasing stress in the back, especially the lower back and neck.

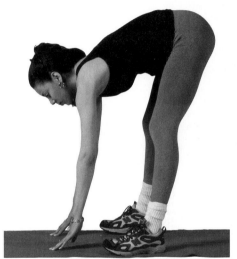

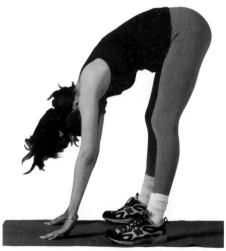

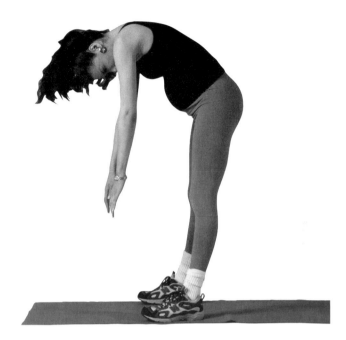

Roll Up—Starting from the forward bend position, roll up vertebra by vertebra lifting your head up last. Be sure to keep your neck released until your back is straight. Women six or more months pregnancy should try not to bend over as far.

Benefit: stretches the back muscles and helps to regain balance.

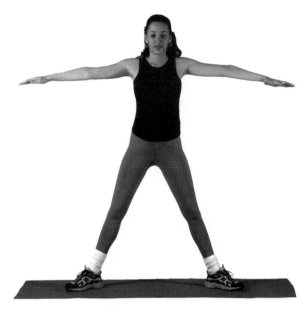

Plies—Stand in a turned out position, legs three feet apart with arms out to the side and at shoulder level. As you bend your knees over your feet, concentrate on stretching you inner thighs, and drop your arms down to the side. As you straighten your legs, lift your arms parallel to the ground. Repeat five times.

Benefit: tones the thighs, adds flexibility to the hip sockets, and relieves tightness in the lower back.

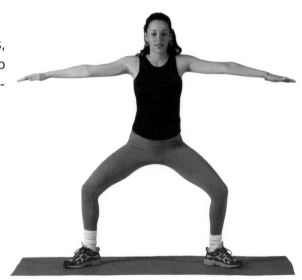

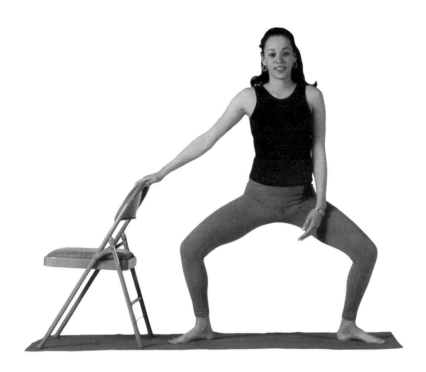

Plies With Chair—Hold lightly onto a chair with one hand for balance. Turn out your legs so that your knees bend over your feet. Concentrate on distributing your weight evenly over both feet. Lift your chest and drop your shoulders. Bend and straighten your knees over your feet, keeping your feet turned out.

Benefit: strengthens the hips, tones pelvic floor and inner thigh muscles.

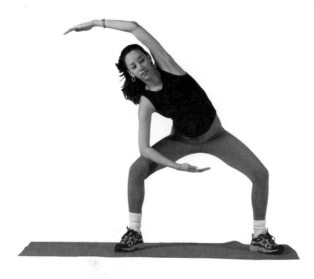

Side Stretch Plies—Stand in a turned out plie position, with knees bent over your feet. Lean your right elbow on your right thigh, and stretch your left arm overhead close to your ear. Take two to three deep breaths and repeat on the other side.

Benefit: tones waist, hips and the thighs, while stretching the inner thighs.

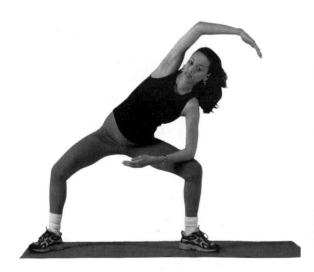

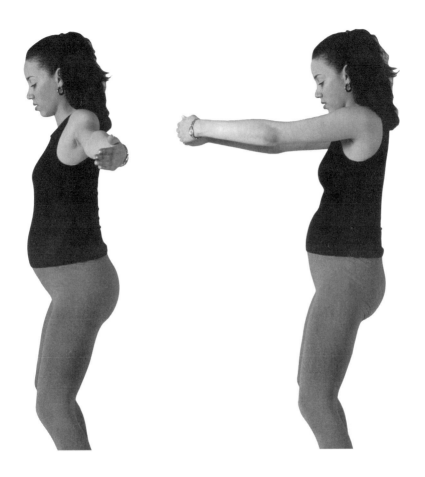

Standing Pelvic Tilt—Stand with your legs hips-width apart. Bend your knees slightly and tilt your pelvis as you bring your arms forward. Return to center and arch slightly. In the third trimester, just tilt–do not arch. Repeat five times.

Benefit: tones hips and buttocks, releases the lower back, and strengthens the pelvic floor and lower abdomen.

Triangle—Stand with your feet three to four feet apart. Turn your left foot in slightly and your right foot out. Line up your right heel with the arch of your left foot. Balance your weight between your feet and hold your arms out to the side, parallel to the ground.

Benefit: great for posture, good for spinal alignment, and an important base for other yoga exercises.

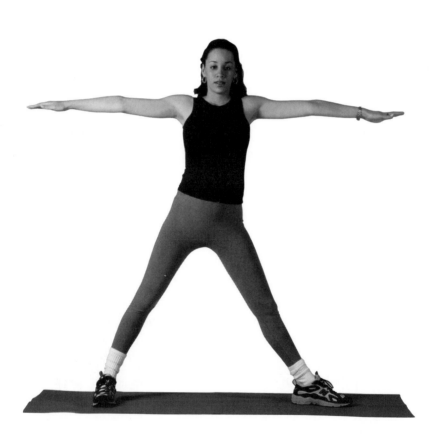

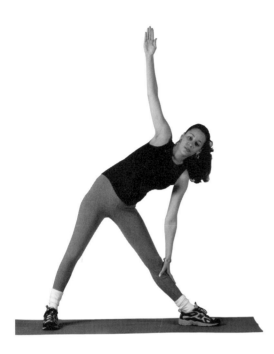

Triangle Lift and Tilt—Get into the triangle pose with your right leg turned out. Tilt your torso to the right (from your pelvis all the way up your spine). Rest your right hand on your right shin. Breathe, keeping your ribcage and pelvis in alignment. Tilt your head up to look at your left hand and down to look at your right hand. Slide back up to center slowly and repeat on the other side.

Benefit: tones the sides of the body, helps improve posture and increases circulation in the hips.

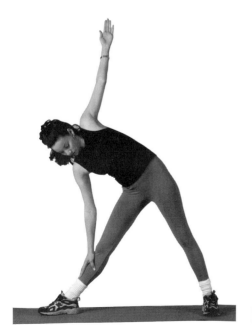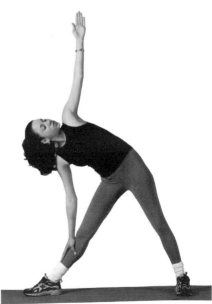

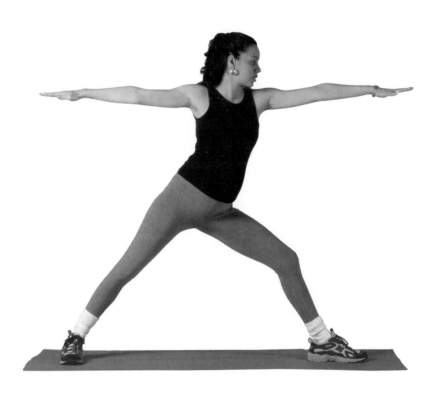

Warrior—From the triangle pose, turn your right leg out and your left leg slightly in. Bend your right knee, keeping your right thigh parallel to the ground. Hold your arms up to the side, parallel to the ground. Lengthen your neck and drop your shoulders. Breathe in and out through your nose smoothly. Switch sides.

Benefit: increases self-confidence and inner strength, strengthens hips and thighs.

Warrior Side Stretch—Get into the warrior pose and lean your right elbow on your thigh. Reach your left arm over your head toward your ear. Take three breaths and return your torso back to center before switching sides.

Benefit: tones the lower abdominals and hips, releases tension from the shoulders.

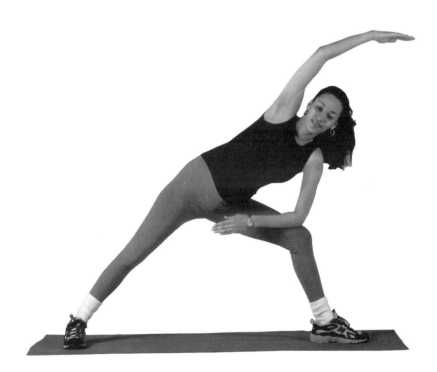

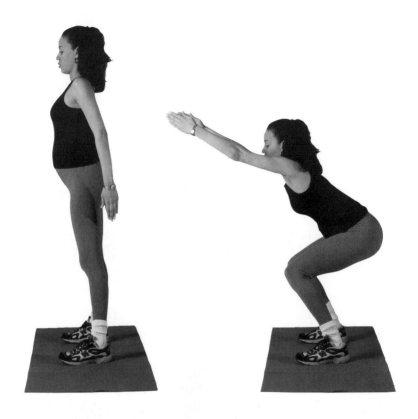

Squat—Stand with your legs hips-width apart. Bend your knees while raising your arms overhead. Keep your back long, from your tailbone to the top of your neck. Inhale as you stand and exhale as you squat. Repeat three times.

Benefit: tones the thighs, helps with balance, adds flexibility and strength to the hips and all the pelvic muscles.

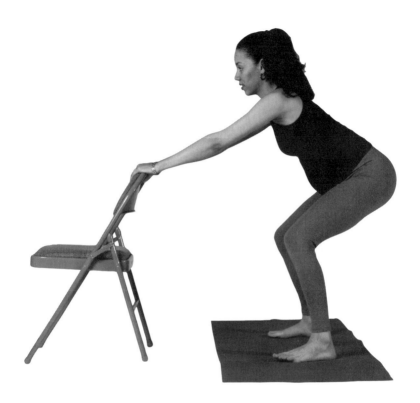

Squat With Chair—Stand with your feet slightly wider then hips-width apart. Bend your knees and drop your hips down. Keep your knees bent over your feet and your back lengthened. Maintain the natural curves of your back, without exaggerating them. Go in and out of the squat three times. Take a baby breath each time you are in the squat.

Benefit: great preparation for labor, strengthens the thighs.

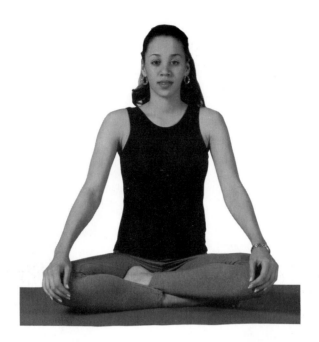

Kegels—The pelvic floor muscles, located between the pubic bone and sacrum, include the birth canal. During pregnancy, with the growing uterus and impending birth, these muscles have added importance. They help support the additional weight and are most important during labor. When you lift them, it is a similar sensation to holding the bladder. Contract and release the pelvic floor muscles, doing a set of twenty.

Elevator Kegels Variation—Contract your pelvic floor muscles up in stages, thinking of the floors in an elevator (first, second, third and fourth). At the top hold your breath, then exhale as you slowly release the contraction, going down the elevator (fourth, third, second, first and basement) giving your pelvic floor a push. Practice as many times a day as you like. The elevator kegel can be done sitting in the cross-legged position, squatting, standing, lying on your side or sitting in a chair.

Benefit: tones the pelvic floor muscles, can make birth and postpartum easier.

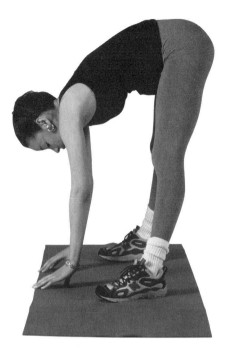

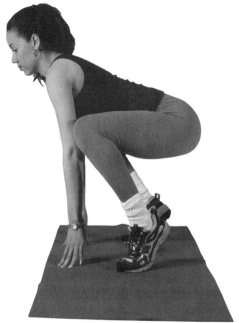

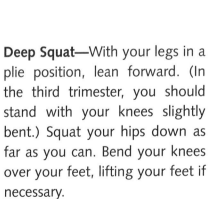

Deep Squat—With your legs in a plie position, lean forward. (In the third trimester, you should stand with your knees slightly bent.) Squat your hips down as far as you can. Bend your knees over your feet, lifting your feet if necessary.

Benefit: great for all the joints of the legs, very good for circulation, and good for labor preparation.

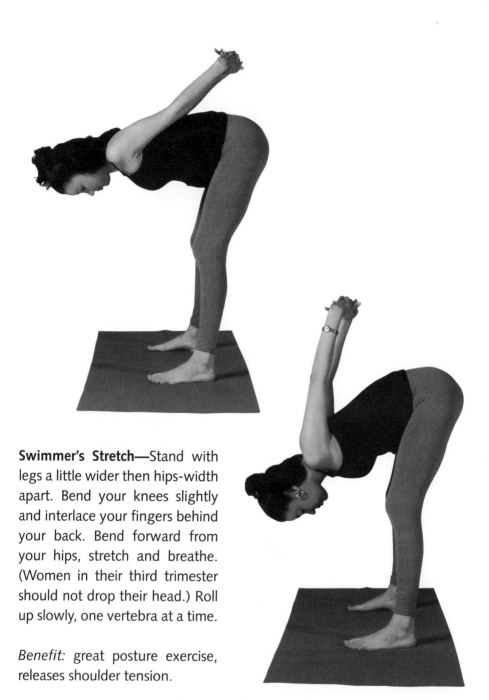

Swimmer's Stretch—Stand with legs a little wider then hips-width apart. Bend your knees slightly and interlace your fingers behind your back. Bend forward from your hips, stretch and breathe. (Women in their third trimester should not drop their head.) Roll up slowly, one vertebra at a time.

Benefit: great posture exercise, releases shoulder tension.

Prayer Pose—Stand with your feet pointed forward and your legs hips-width apart. Bring your palms together in front of your chest. Tune into your breathing as you close your eyes for a moment.

Benefit: helps to center your emotions and calm your nerves.

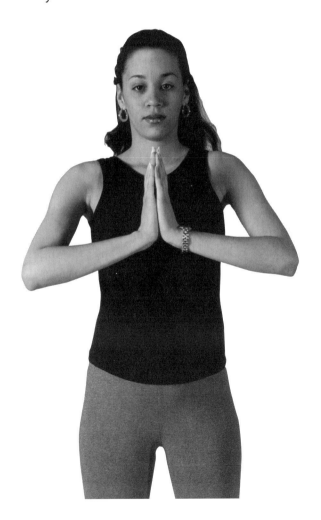

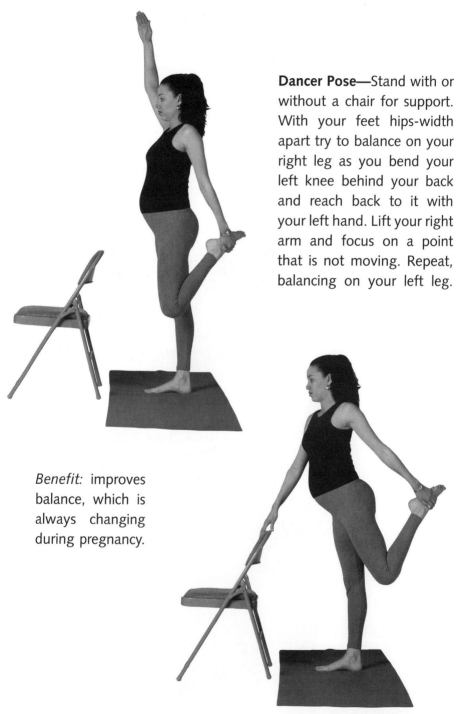

Dancer Pose—Stand with or without a chair for support. With your feet hips-width apart try to balance on your right leg as you bend your left knee behind your back and reach back to it with your left hand. Lift your right arm and focus on a point that is not moving. Repeat, balancing on your left leg.

Benefit: improves balance, which is always changing during pregnancy.

Tree Pose—Balance on your left leg, turning your right leg out. Bring the sole of your right foot up to your inner left leg, either under the knee or above it. Raise your left arm toward the sky. Breathe and repeat on the other side.

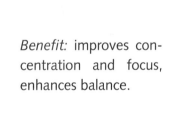

Benefit: improves concentration and focus, enhances balance.

51

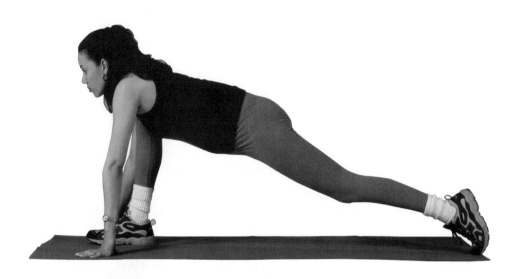

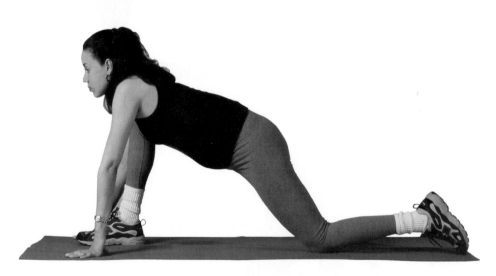

Lunge—Begin with your feet together. Lunge your right leg all the way back, keeping your hips low and gazing slightly forward. Bend and straighten your right knee three times. Repeat on other side.

Benefit: stretches the front of the thigh, ankles and shins.

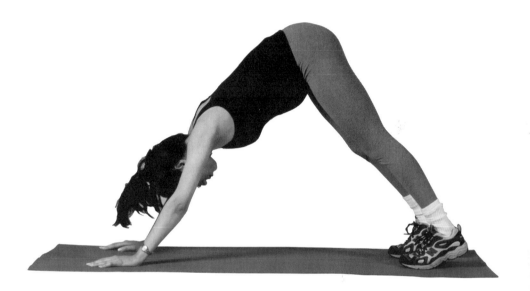

Down Dog—From the lunge bring both legs back. Press your palms flat down and lift your hips high in the air. Stretch your hamstrings, and press your back heels down on the floor. Take three breaths.

Benefit: strengthens the shoulders and upper back, releases the hamstrings.

Bent Knee Down Dog—From the down dog position, slightly bend your knees and straighten and lengthen from your arms up to your hips.

Benefit: releases the lower back and hips.

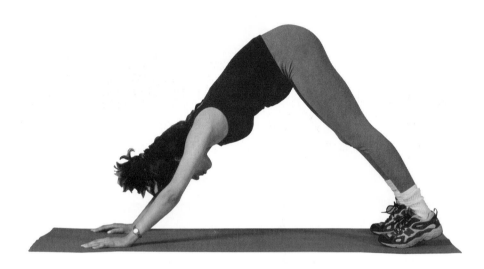

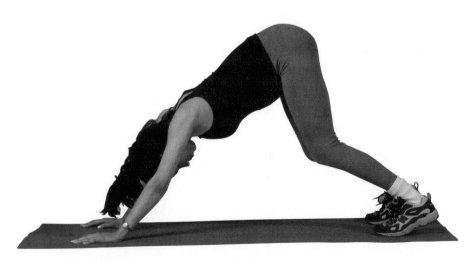

ON HANDS AND KNEES

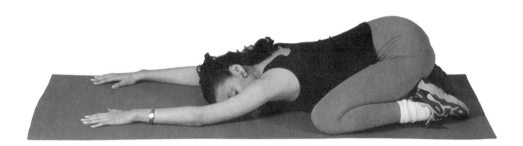

Child Pose—On all fours, slide your hips back to your heels. Adjust your knees so that your belly has room to comfortably rest between your knees. Stretch your arms out in front of you. Release your neck muscles and breath smoothly.

Benefit: releases tension in the lower back and shoulders, aids digestion.

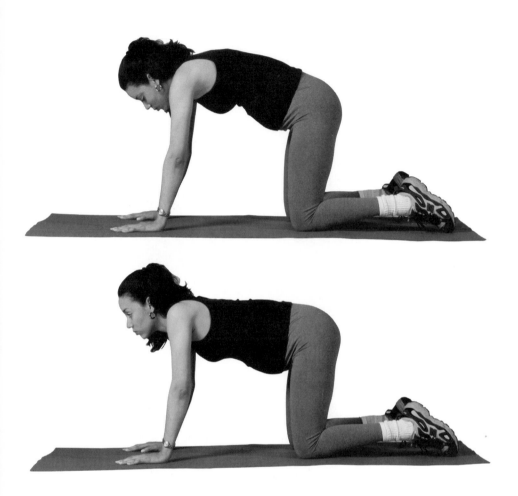

Cat Pose—On your hands and knees, with your hands shoulder-width apart and your knees hips-width apart, feel the length of your back from your tailbone through your neck. Round your back as you exhale and arch your back as you inhale (arch very little in the last trimester). Repeat five to ten times. Only do what is comfortable for you.

Benefit: releases tension in the back, balances the nervous system, integrates proper breathing techniques.

56

SIDE & PELVIS EXERCISES

All side leg exercises should be done on one side of the body, before switching to the opposite side to repeat.

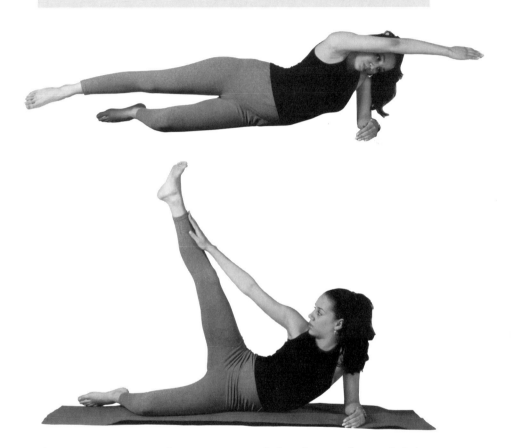

Side Arm to Leg Stretch—Lie on your left side. Bend your left knee and rest on your left elbow. Reach your right arm overhead, keeping your right leg slightly behind you. Inhale. Exhale and touch your right hand to your right ankle. Repeat three to five times. As you progress in your pregnancy, you may want to slightly bend your right knee.

Benefit: tones waist and external obliques, tones the hips, stretches the hamstrings.

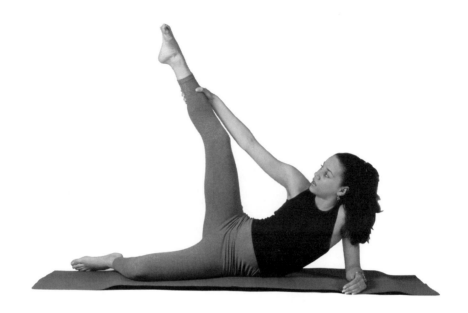

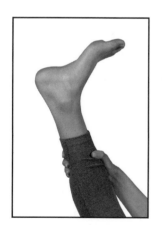 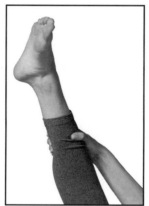 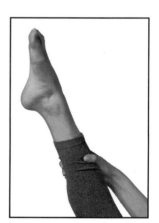

Side Ankle Rotations—Lie on your left side. Raise your right foot in the air and rotate your ankles three times in each direction. Switch sides.

Benefit: increases circulation in the feet, ankles and the calves, decreases swelling in the ankles.

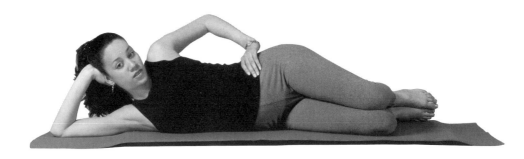

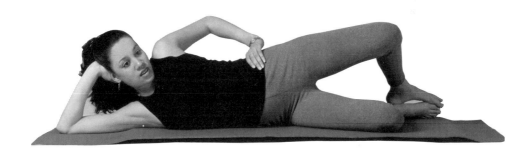

Side Knee Lifts—Lie on your right side. Comfortably rest your head in your hand and keep both knees bent, hips facing forward. With your feet touching, raise and lower your left knee five to ten times. Switch sides.

Benefit: tones the sides of the hips, stretches the inner thighs, tightens the buttocks muscles.

Hip Shaper—Lie on your right side. Comfortably rest your head in your hand. With both knees bent, bring your left foot to your right knee, then your knee to your foot. Repeat two to five times. Switch sides.

Benefit: tones the small muscles of the outer hip, which will help you get back in shape easier after the baby arrives.

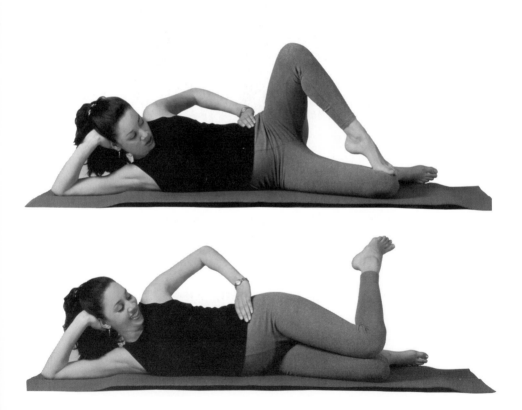

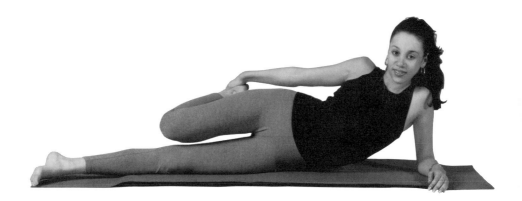

Lying Quadriceps Stretch—Lie on your right side. Bend your left knee back and hold onto your left ankle. Hold for a count of five breaths. Switch sides.

Benefit: stretches the quadriceps and shoulders.

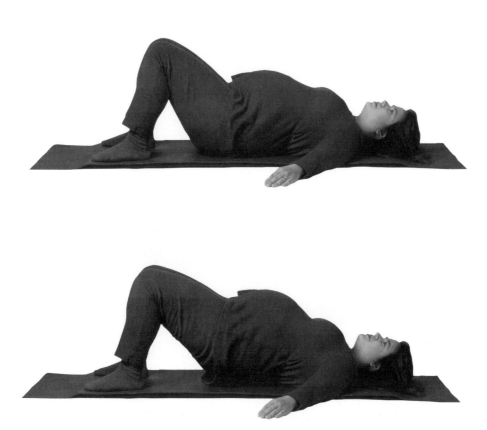

Mini Pelvic Tilts—Lie on your mat, arms down by your side. Tighten your hips and tilt your lower back off the ground as you exhale. Repeat five times.

Benefit: alleviates tiredness in the lower back, and strengthens the pelvic floor.

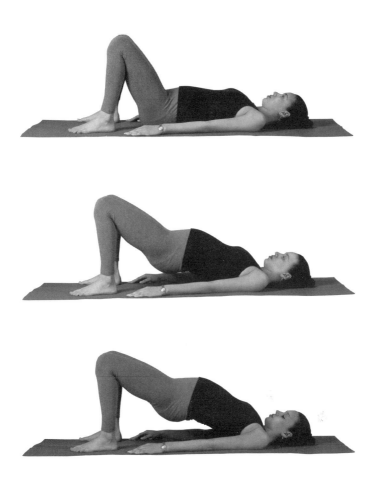

Pelvic Tilt—Lie on your mat, with your knees bent and your spine touching the mat. Relax your neck. Your feet should be hips-width apart (slightly further apart as you reach the third trimester). Slowly tighten your buttocks and lift your spine vertebra by vertebra. Roll up until your weight rests along the top of your shoulders. Take a full breath. Then slowly roll down your spine. Repeat up to three times.

Benefit: great for releasing tension in the spine and shoulders, and tunes into the stomach muscles.

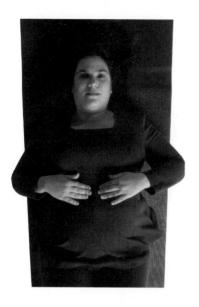 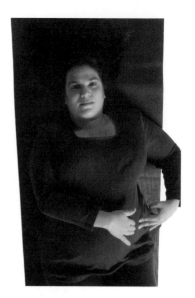

Pelvic Clock—Tilt your pelvis, rock to your right hip, arch your lower back, and rock to your left hip. Then, make a complete circle to the right three times. Reverse and make three circles to the left.

Benefit: relieves lower back tension.

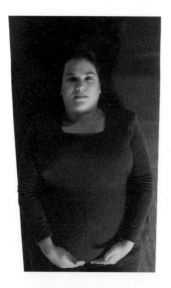 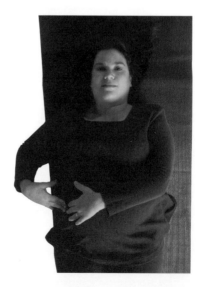

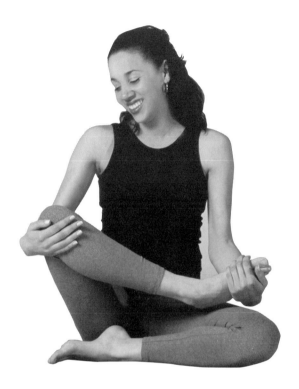

Tailor Stretch—Sit cross-legged, lift your right knee and ankle and rotate in the hip socket back and forth three times. Return and repeat on the other side.

Benefit: articulates the hip sockets, increasing circulation and flexibility in the pelvic region.

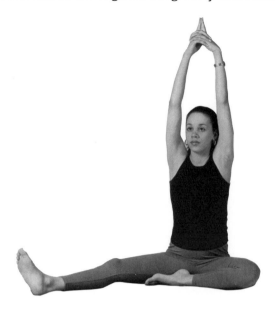

Hurdler Stretch—Sit on your hip sockets with your right leg extended slightly out to the side. Reach both arms overhead and inhale. Drop your arms and head down, exhale. Hold and take a baby breath. Stretch your right arm down to your shin, keeping your left arm by your ear. Breathe fully. Repeat on the other side.

Benefit: releases tightness in the back and hamstrings, tones the waist.

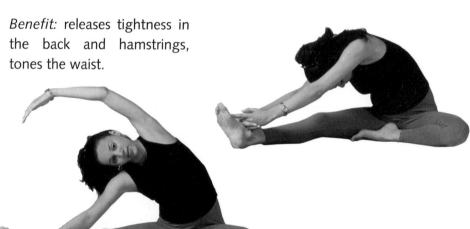

By stretching and gently toning the waist muscles in many of these exercises you will maintain tone even as your stomach grows during pregnancy. Although it may seem as if you will never get your waist back, these exercises might help you to actually end up with a smaller waistline than before your pregnancy!

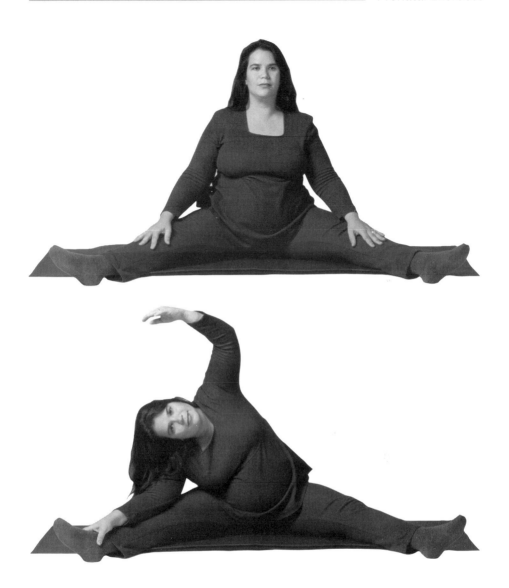

Straddle Side Stretch—Sit evenly on your sit bones, stretch to the left side with your left arm on your shin and your right arm in the air. Breathe and return to center. Stretch to the other side.

Benefit: stretches the inner thighs, tones your waist, great for the pelvic floor muscles.

PART V – POSTNATAL EXERCISES

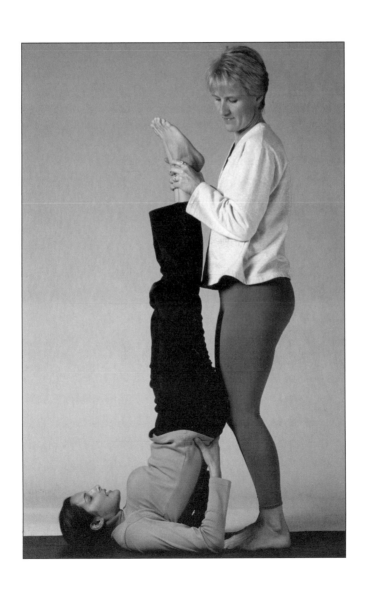

It is important to do yoga and other forms of exercise after you deliver your baby. Taking care of yourself is essential now that you are taking care of your baby. Daily gentle exercise including yoga can help restore your muscle strength. Yoga helps you return to the shape you were in before pregnancy. In the beginning it may seem overwhelming. You're adjusting to having a new baby. Everyone's sleeping schedule is off. Your hormones are readjusting. You may be nursing.

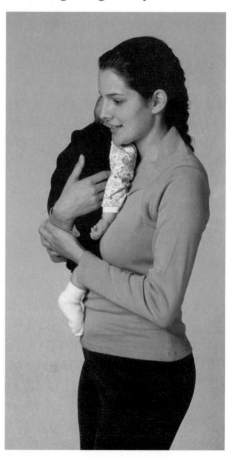

Most women who deliver naturally can move around a little and perform small tasks the day after they give birth. After a few days, some women can walk normally, depending on whether they've had an episiotomy. If you have had a caesarean section or complicated birth, check with your doctor before starting an exercise program. Most women can perform the following yoga exercises a few days after delivery: belly breathing, pelvic tilts, foot circles, kegels, and more.

Check for Dialysis Rectus after you have given birth. The third trimester is often a time when this can occur. If dialysis has occurred, wrap your hands (or a towel) around your ribs as you do abdominal curls.

After delivery, many women are eager to resume their pre-pregnancy routine. According to the American College of Obstetricians and Gynecologists, many physiologic and morphologic changes persist four to six weeks post-partum. Be aware that it usually takes nine months for the body to totally return to normal. Much depends on whether you nurse. Nursing can help you lose weight after the baby's birth and also helps the uterus return to its previous size. Expect, however, to keep on five to seven pounds needed for nursing. Those pounds will drop off soon after you stop nursing. You should resume your pre-pregnancy yoga routine gradually, depending on how you are feeling, and only after checking with your doctor.

Starting to do yoga soon after your baby arrives (within the first six weeks) is your way of taking time out to rejuvenate. You can do some yoga with the baby by your side or in your lap. For other routines, it might be more comfortable to place the baby in a bouncer.

You may want to play relaxing music. Place a yoga mat on the floor, make sure the room is a comfortable temperature. Have two medium size pillows available. Find a place at home where you feel comfortable doing your yoga stretches and massage with your child, partner or on your own.

Remember to start out slowly, just trying to do a little yoga each day—even if just for five minutes. Do not feel guilty if you skip a day or two. Simply start again. The yoga will give you back so much. You will breathe more efficiently, your abdominals will be toned, you will release stress and tension. The idea that once you have a baby you never get your body back is a fallacy. If you follow this book and do some cross-training, in about three months you can be in better shape than you were before you got pregnant.

Many of the following exercises can be done with the baby or while nursing, which means that when you want or need to be with your baby, you can still do some yoga.

Horsey Ride—Lie on your back with a pillow under your shoulders. Balance your baby on your shins with his or her face looking down at you. Make eye contact. Rock your knees back and forth gently.

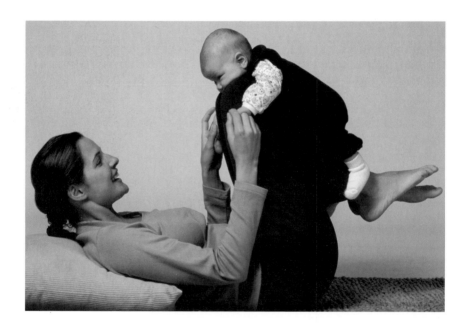

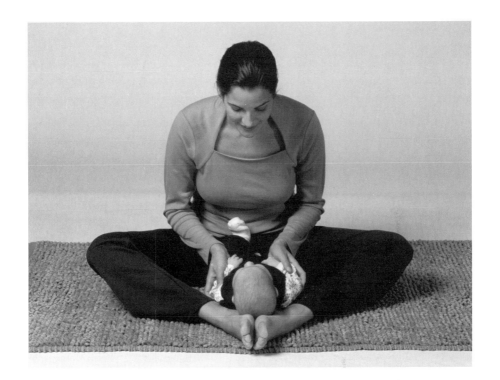

Butterfly Pose—Sit on your sit bones with the soles of your feet together and your legs apart. In the butterfly pose, you can sit with your baby in front of you either on a pillow or resting on your legs.

Benefit: improves posture, relaxes lower back, tones hips, and bonds with baby.

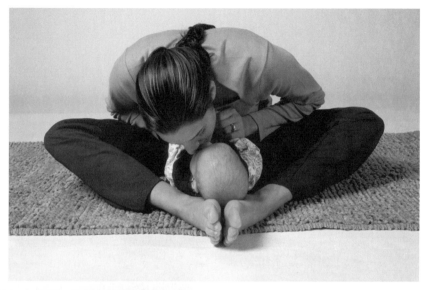

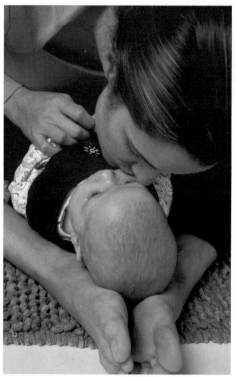

Kiss in Butterfly Pose—While sitting in the butterfly pose, lean forward to kiss your baby. This exercise gives you incentive to stretch a little further and is a great inner thigh stretch.

Benefit: releases tension in the pelvis and lower back.

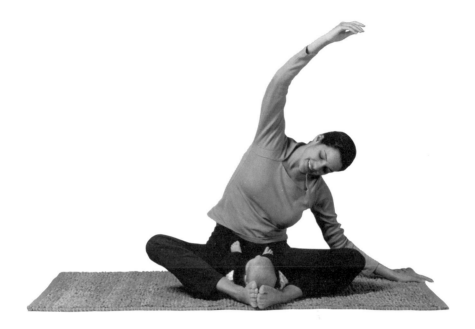

Seated Side Stretch—In the butterfly pose with baby between your legs, exhale as you stretch to the side, inhale as you straighten to center. Repeat on opposite side.

Benefit: tones the waist.

Spinal Twist—Sit in the butterfly pose with your baby between your legs, your right hand on the floor by your lower back and your left hand on your right knee. Inhale as you lengthen your back. Exhale as you twist to the right. Take two full breaths. Release and twist in the other direction.

Benefit: balances the nervous system and improves digestion.

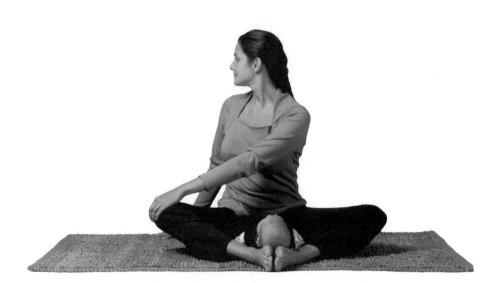

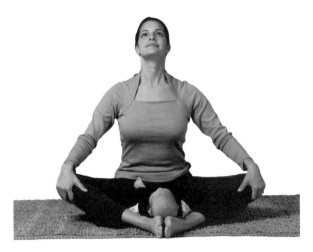
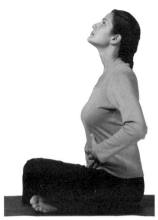
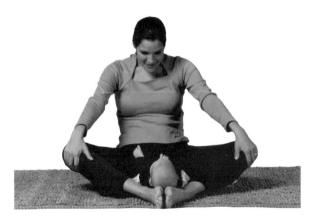
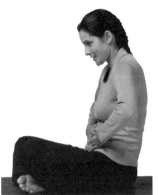

Arch and Round—In the butterfly pose, hold your baby between your legs, placing your hands on your knees. Round and arch your back from the bottom of your spine to the top. Inhale as you arch and exhale as you round.

Benefit: balances the nerves and increases circulation up and down the spine.

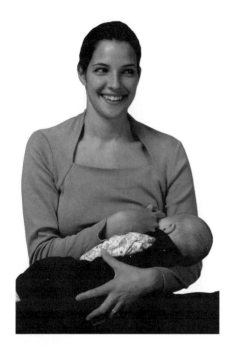

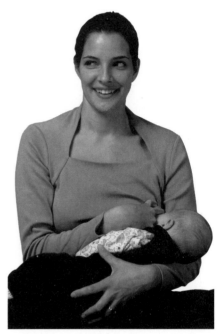

Eye Exercises—Sit cross-legged, drop your shoulders, lift your chest and lengthen your neck. Without moving your head, look all the way up with your eyes, look as far as you can to the right, all the way down, then all the way to the left. Make three complete circles to the right. Rest, and then perform three complete circles to the left. Rest.

Benefit: releases eye tension.

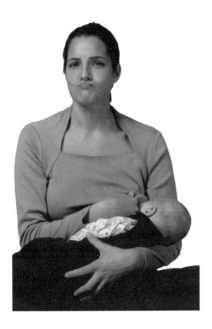 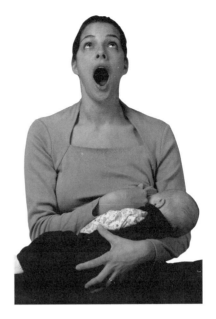

Face Exercises—Open and stretch your mouth to release jaw tightness.

Benefit: releases tension.

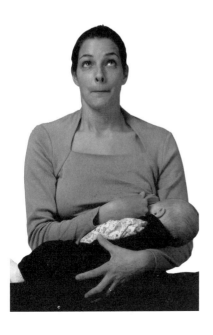 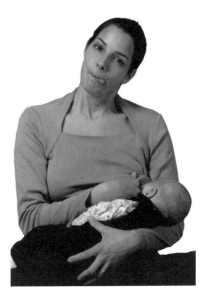

79

Side Neck Stretch—Sitting in the cross-legged position, this exercise can also be done while nursing. Extend your left ear to your left shoulder, and drop your right shoulder. Look down toward the ground and inhale. Look up to sky and exhale. Repeat with your right ear to your right shoulder.

Benefit: stretches the side of the neck and upper shoulder muscles.

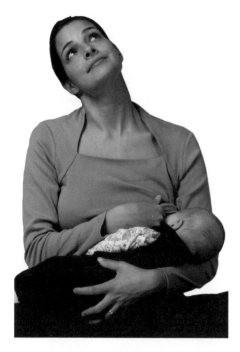

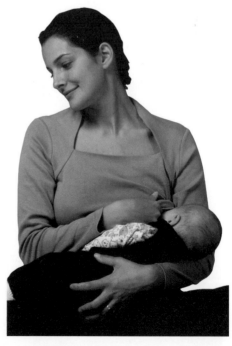

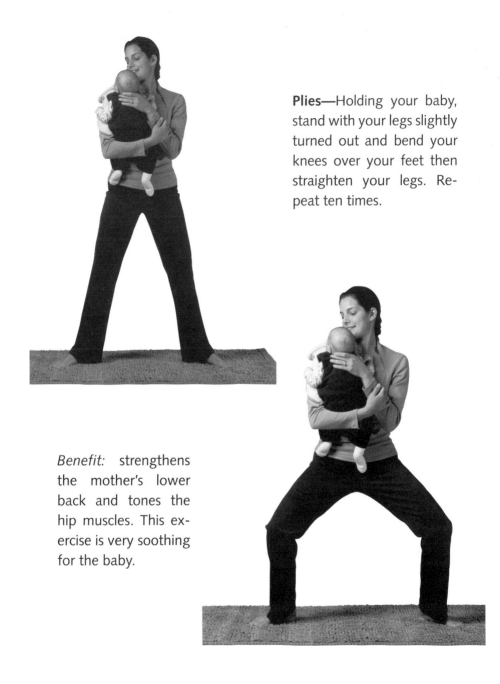

Plies—Holding your baby, stand with your legs slightly turned out and bend your knees over your feet then straighten your legs. Repeat ten times.

Benefit: strengthens the mother's lower back and tones the hip muscles. This exercise is very soothing for the baby.

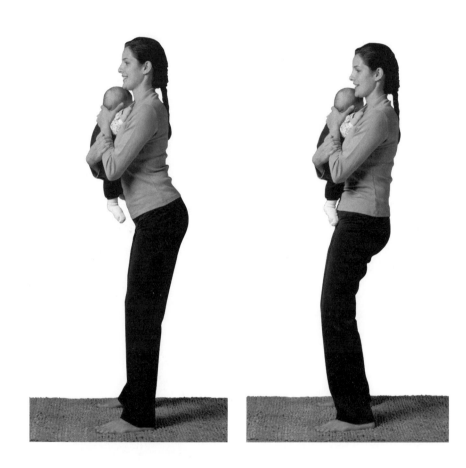

Standing Pelvic Tilt—Holding your baby, bend your knees and slightly tilt your pelvis forward and back.

Benefit: firms buttocks and hips, and releases tightness in the lower back.

Belly Breathing—This exercise can be done on a mat or in a chair. Cross your legs. Place your hands over your stomach. Breathe through your nose unless you are congested. Feel your belly rock forward as you inhale and feel it rock back to your spine as you exhale.

Benefit: tones your stomach muscles and tone the internal organs.

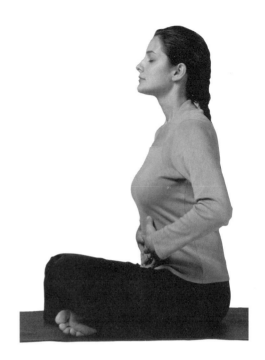

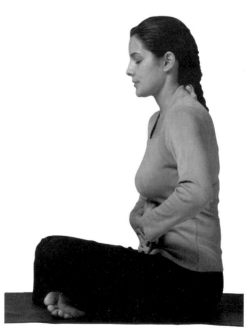

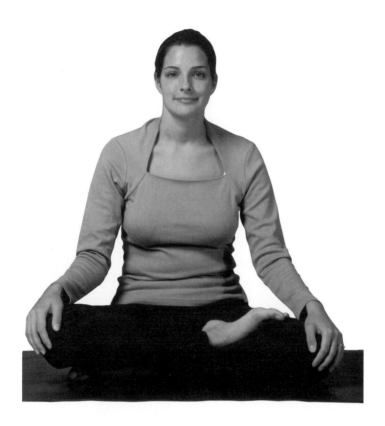

Kegels—The pelvic floor muscles are located in between the pubic bone and sacrum, also including the birth canal. When you lift them it is a similar sensation to holding the bladder. Contract and release the pelvic floor muscles, doing a set of twenty.

Benefit: tones the pelvic floor and abdominal muscles and increases circulation to the pelvic region.

Ankle Rotation—Lie on your back with a pillow under your head. Lift your right leg up rotate your ankle three times in each direction. Repeat. Switch sides.

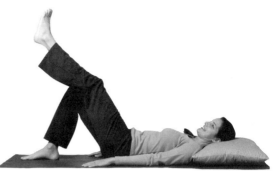

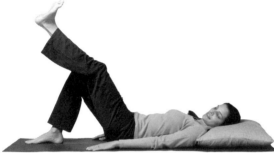

Benefit: warms up the ankles and helps to eliminate water retention.

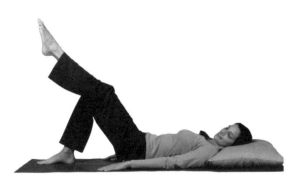

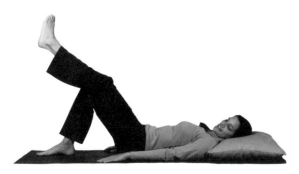

Modified Sit-up—Lie down with your knees bent, hands cradling your head. Exhale as you lift your head, inhale as you lower it. Concentrate on using your lower abdominal muscles.

Benefit: tones the lower abdominal muscles that have been stretched out during pregnancy.

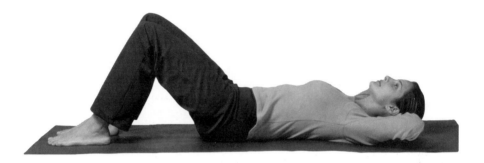

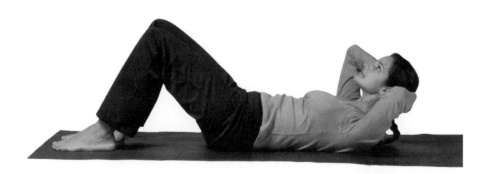

Cross Over—Lie down with your arms over head. Inhale and keep your knees slightly bent. Reach your right hand toward your left leg and exhale. Return back to center and inhale. Repeat on other side.

Benefit: tones the side of the stomach and waist.

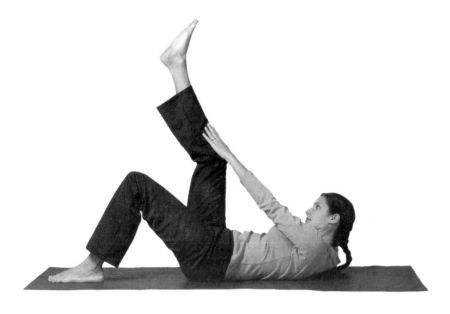

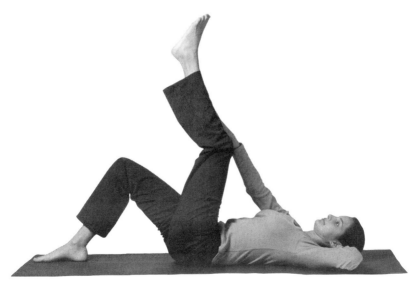

All side leg exercises should be done on one side of the body, before switching to the opposite side to repeat.

Side Leg Lift—Lie on your right side, resting on your elbow with your bottom knee slightly bent. Lift your left leg about a foot and a half off the ground, so the hip does not turn out and the knee remains facing forward. Slowly lower your left leg down to the ground and breathe smoothly. Repeat ten times on both sides.

Benefit: tones the outside of the leg and hip.

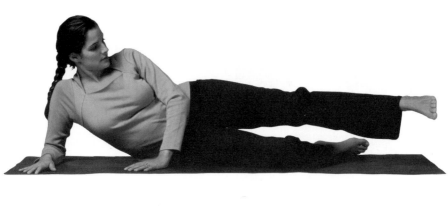

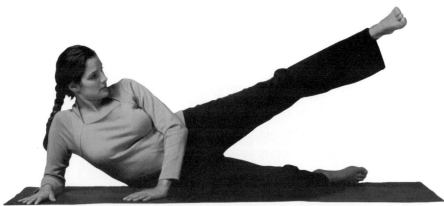

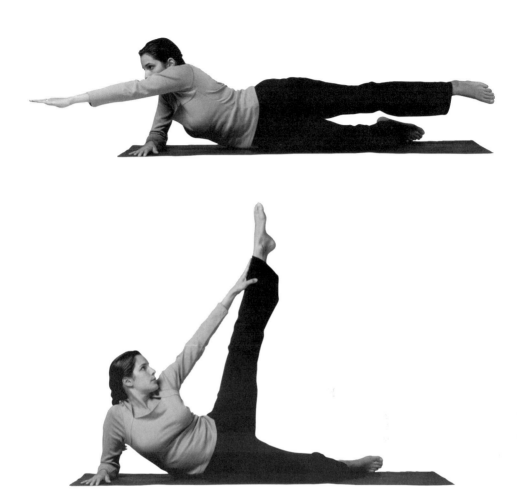

Modified Leg Lifts—Lie on your right side, resting on your elbow with your bottom knee slightly bent. Reach your left arm overhead while stretching your left leg slightly in back of you and inhale. On the exhale, bring your left foot to your left hand. Repeat three times. Then, proceed to the knee lift on this side before changing leg position.

Benefit: stretches and tones waist and hips.

Side Knee Lift—Lie on your right side with knees bent and feet touching. Stabilize your hips, raising and lowering your left knee ten times. Repeat on other side.

Benefit: tones the hips.

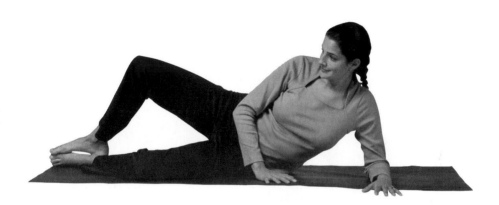

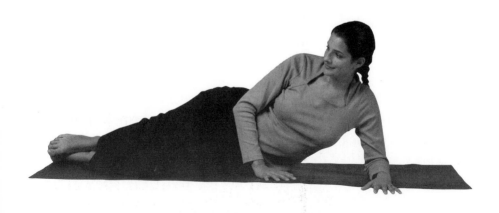

Inner Thigh Lift—Lie on your right side, bending your left leg behind your right thigh. Lift and lower your right leg five to ten times. Repeat on other side.

Benefit: excellent for toning the inner thigh.

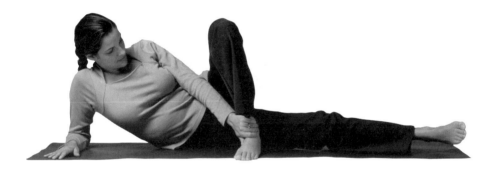

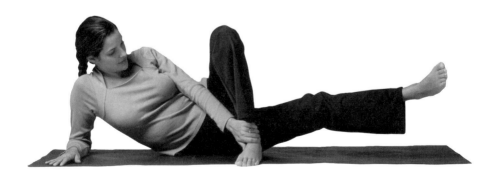

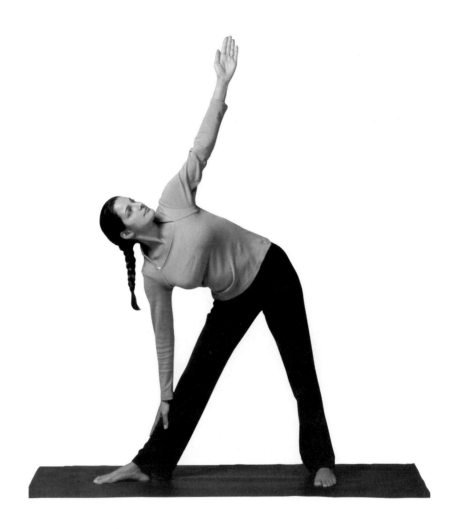

Triangle Side Stretch—Assume the triangle pose and tilt back from the tailbone, moving your entire back and not just your waist. Slide your right hand down your right shin and stretch your left arm to the sky.

Benefit: tones the waist, hips, thighs, and backs of legs, and improves balance and posture.

Warrior—From the triangle pose, turn your right leg out and your left leg slightly in. Bend your right knee, keeping your right thigh parallel to the ground. Hold your arms up to the side, parallel to the ground. Lengthen your neck and drop your shoulders. Breathe in and out through your nose smoothly. Switch sides.

Benefit: increases feeling strong mentally and physically.

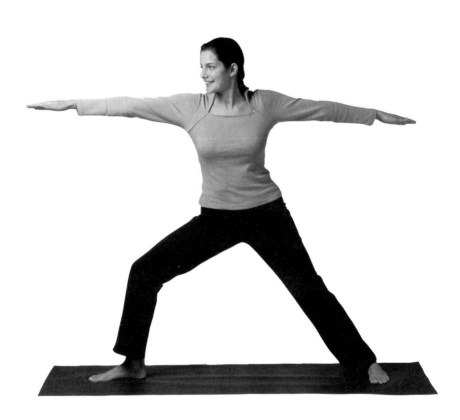

Lunge—Repeat regular lunge adjusting hip width for comfort.

Benefit: strong stretch for the quads and lower abdominals.

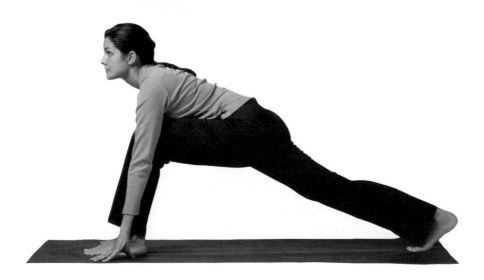

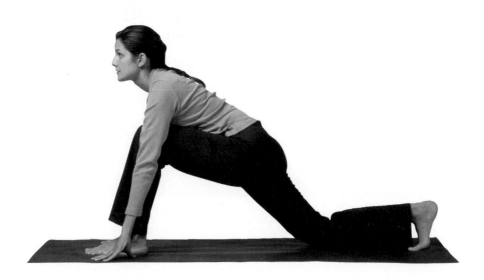

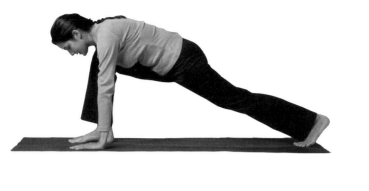

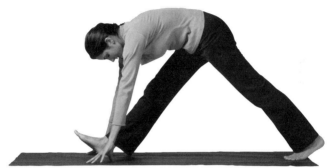

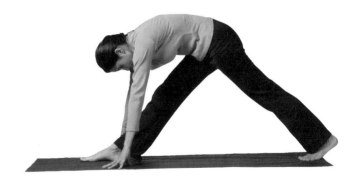

Lunge Variation—Straighten your front leg as much as you can, balancing on your fingertips and flexing your ankle.

Benefit: gives a more intense stretch to the hamstrings and calf muscles.

95

Half Moon Back Bend—Stand with feet hips-width apart or together. Tighten your buttocks and arch your upper back, extending your arms overhead and by your ears. Breathe fully.

Benefit: releases tension in the upper back, tones the waist.

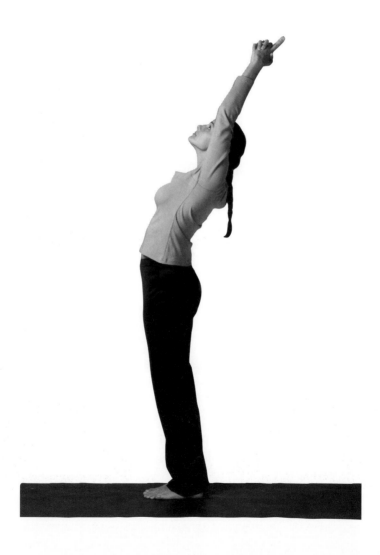

Triangle Spinal Twist—Stand in a triangle pose with your right leg turned out, left leg turned slightly in and your weight is evenly distributed. Your arms should be parallel to the ground. Twist your upper body toward the right and bend from your hips until your torso is parallel to the ground. Lift your right arm up in the air. Continue the twist through your spine. Breathe evenly. Gaze back or to the sky. It feels great to twist after you have had the baby. Repeat on other side.

Benefit: tones the organs and relieves tired backs.

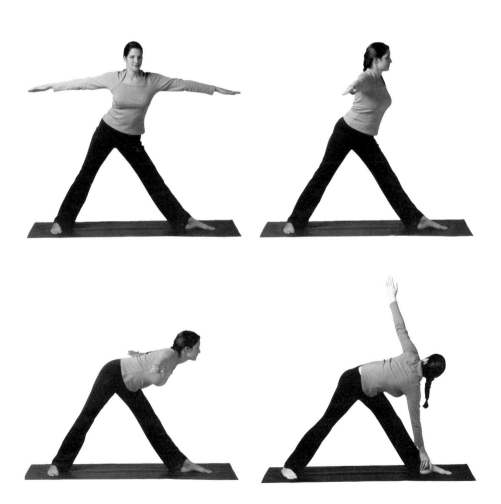

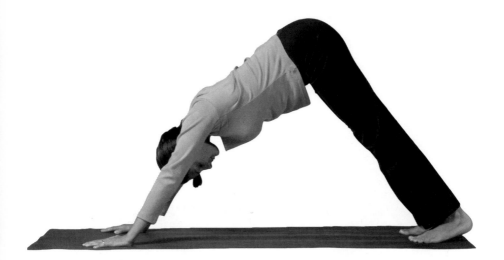

Down Dog—Similar to prenatal down dog, but now you can place your feet closer together. You also can hold the pose for three full breaths. When you are pregnant you hold for a shorter time.

Benefit: strengthens the upper back and shoulders that need to be strong to carry and nurse the baby.

Plank Pose—Hold your body parallel to the ground. Contract your abdominals and back muscles to keep your body straight. Breathe. A variation of this exercise is the bent knee plank pose, which puts less stress on the lower back.

Benefit: tones arms and stomach muscles.

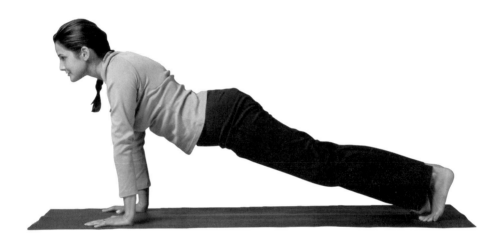

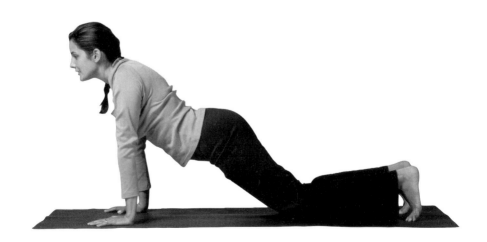

Up Dog—From the plank pose hold your arms out straight and point your toes. Let your hips drop toward the ground.

Benefit: increases circulation in the torso, tones shoulders and arms.

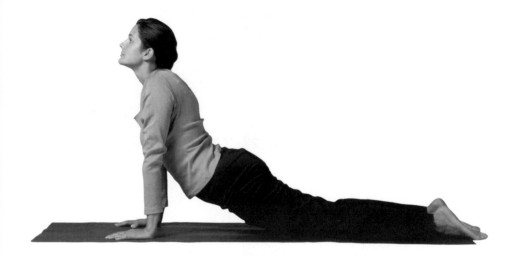

Cat Pose—Similar to the prenatal version of pose, but you can arch your back fully. Inhale as you arch your back. Exhale as you pull your abdominals in and round your back. Repeat five times.

Benefit: relieves lower back pain.

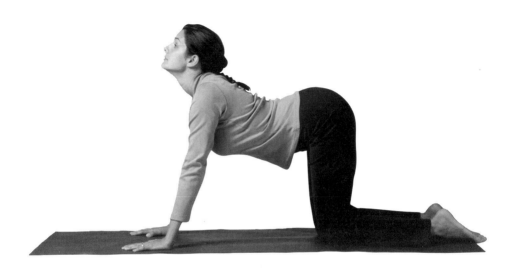

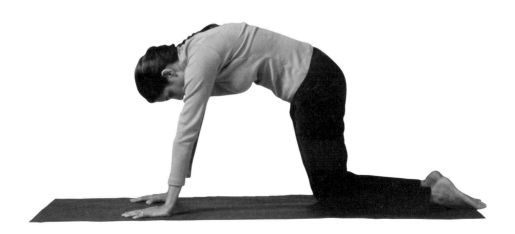

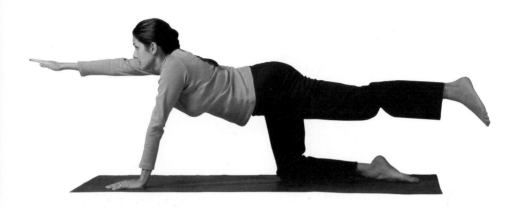

Cat Stretch—From the cat pose, inhale, reach your right arm up in front of you while lifting your left leg behind you. Exhale. Return to the cat pose and inhale as you reach your left arm up and lift your right leg back.

Benefit: balances the nerves.

Cat Side Kicks—From the cat pose, lift and lower your right knee out to the side. Keep your knee bent with both the knee and foot on the same level. Repeat five to ten times on each side.

Benefit: firms the outer thigh muscles.

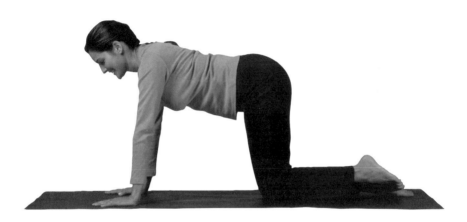

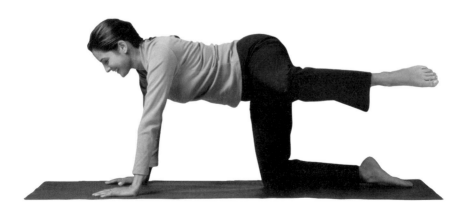

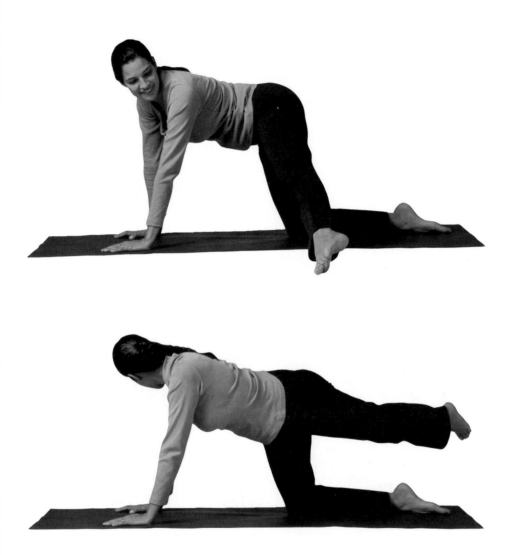

Cat Twist—From cat stretch, extend your right leg to the side. Keeping it straight swing it to the left side. Start with your foot slightly off the floor. Progress to foot at hip's height. Let your head follow. Do five times and repeat on other side.

Benefit: tones the waist and hips, increases overall circulation.

Cobra—Lie on your stomach with your chin on the mat, and your feet touching or hips-width apart. Lift your head and upper torso off the ground, keeping your elbows close to your sides. Lengthen your neck and look at a point in front of you on the floor. Breathe smoothly.

Benefit: strengthens your lower back and balances the muscles up and down the back.

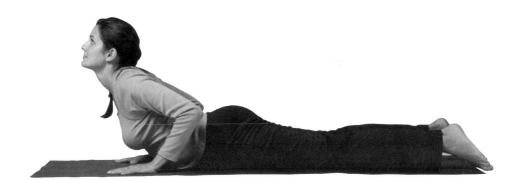

Child Pose—Begin on your hands and knees, with your knees hips width apart. Reach your hips back toward your heels, extending your arms out in front of you or behind you with your head to one side.

Benefit: re-energizing after workout, releases the lower back, helps relieve gas and constipation, and is good for overall relaxation.

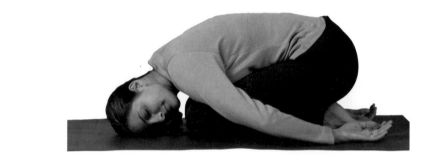

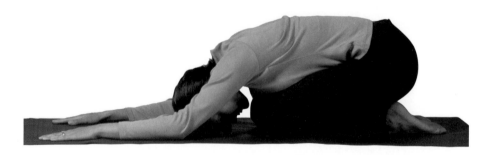

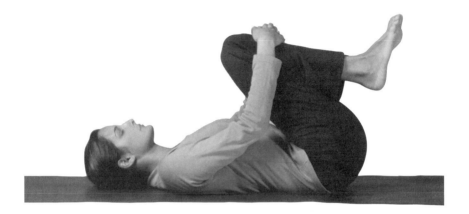

Knees to Chest—Lie on the mat with your knees bent and relax your neck. Gently pull your knees in toward you.

Benefit: releases the lower back.

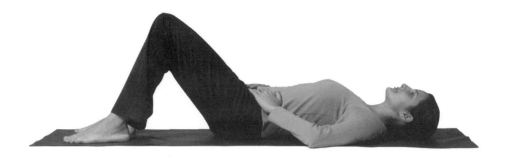

Mini-Pelvic Tilt—Lie on a mat with your knees bent and your feet hips-width apart. Tilt your pelvis, lifting your lower back off the ground as you exhale. Release your lower back down to the floor as you inhale. Repeat five times.

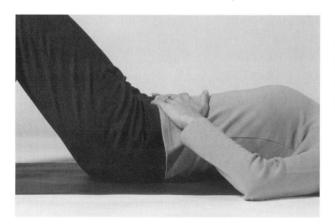

Benefit: relaxes the lower back and helps to tone the pelvic floor and hip muscles.

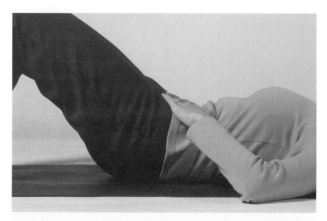

Pelvic Tilt—Lie on your back with your knees parallel to hips. Tilt your pelvis up to the ceiling. Interlace the fingers under your hips.

Benefit: strengthens the back and the front of the shoulders.

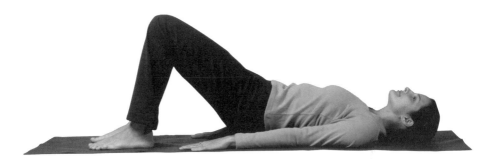

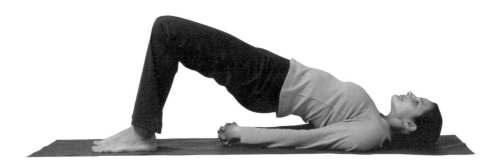

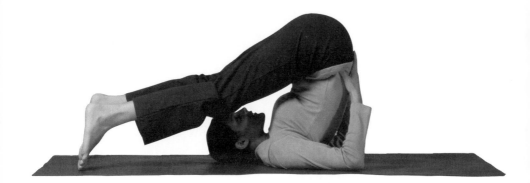

Plow—Lie on your back. Slowly roll your feet over your head until your toes touch the floor behind you. If more comfortable, you can bend your knees to the floor instead. Do not turn your head from side to side and support your back by placing your hands on your lower back with finger tips reaching to your hips.

Benefit: prepares you for shoulder stand.

Shoulder Stand—Supporting your back with your hands, lift your legs up into the air. Feel the weight distributed across the top of your shoulders. Do not turn your neck while in the pose.

Benefit: Good pose for the glands and balances the hormones.

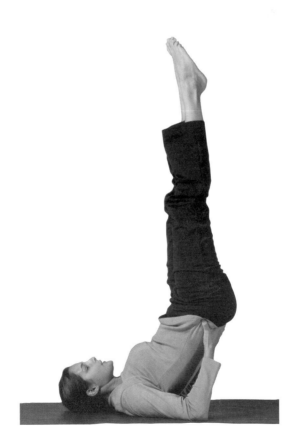

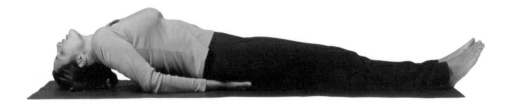

Fish—Lie on your mat. Lean on your elbows and arch your back, gently touching the top of your head to the ground. Stick out your tongue.

Benefit: good balance pose to do after the shoulder stand and balances the thyroid gland.

PART VI – DOUBLE YOGA

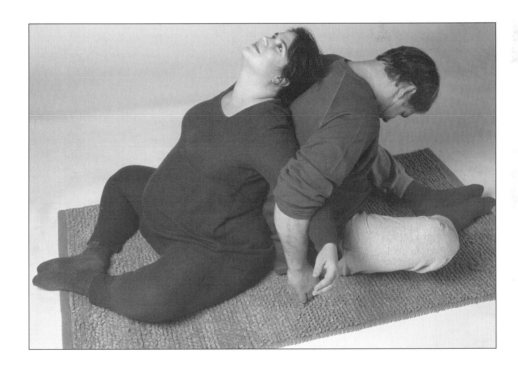

Yoga helps to restore the balance between body and mind. By practicing yoga the body become more supple, sensitive and energized, allowing the mind to reach full potential with less stress. Although yoga originated thousands of years ago, double yoga is an exciting new branch of yoga that you do with a partner. It is a great way to bond and relax together.

Although pregnancy is a very special time for the mother, it is also a very exciting time for the father. By practicing double yoga with you, the father can feel more included in the excitement of the pregnancy and birth, and you both become more sensitive to each other's needs. Since pregnancy is a time when both the woman and the man can feel anxious, doing the breathing exercises together will help relieve physical and mental stress.

When you practice yoga with a partner, you pull against each other gently and increase your stretch. Both partners can tune into what feels tight, achy and tired, and you can help each other.

There is an energy exchange when two people hold yoga poses together. Simply sitting back to back and tuning into the baby breath is a wonderful way to relax together. You might want to sit in this position and practice the Guided Relaxation in Part X.

The combined energy of two people working together enables you to experience the pose differently that when doing yoga alone. You may find that you have better concentration and that certain positions are easier to hold.

Many subtle lessons in your relationship with your partner are demonstrated through double yoga. You learn how to communicate better non-verbally. I also encourage couples to talk about their experience of certain poses. Breathe, communicate and enjoy stretching together. These skills will help you throughout pregnancy and labor.

DOUBLE YOGA POSITIONS

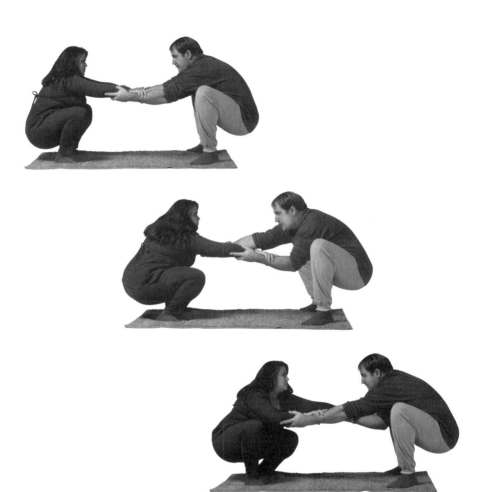

Suspension Bridge—Stand facing each other (about four to five feet apart), with your feet wider then hips-width apart. Hold hands. Bend your knees slightly as you lean away from each other, turning out your legs slightly and lowering into a squat. Push and pull gently with one arm and then the other. Reverse the pose slowly.

Benefit: lengthens the back and stretches the shoulders.

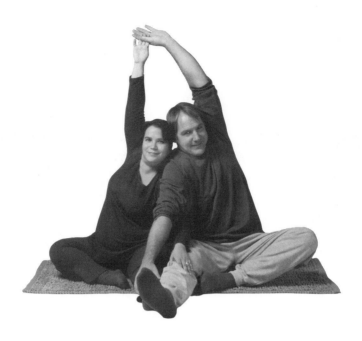

Hurdler—Sit with your right hip against your partner's left hip and your left leg bent. Reach your right arm down your right leg and lift your left arm up in the air (reverse for your partner). Take three long breaths.

Benefit: relaxes and tones the torso and back.

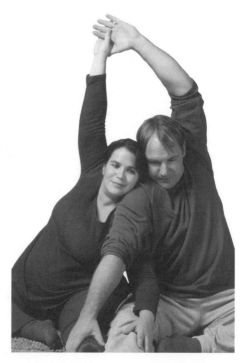

116

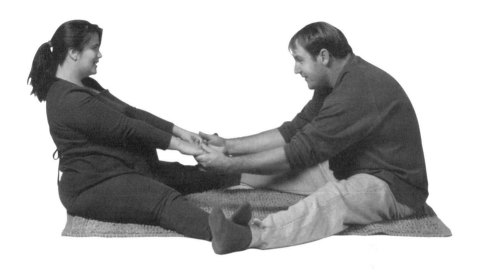

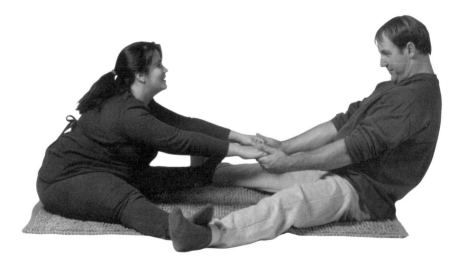

Straddle—Sit face to face with legs wide apart. The partner with the shorter legs places them on the inside. Your partner stretches you forward as he leans back. Then, pull your partner forward as you lean back. Repeat three times.

Benefit: stretches inner thighs, releases tension in the hips and shoulders.

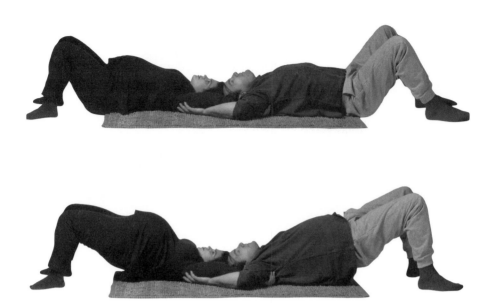

Double Bridge—Lie head to head feet facing away from each other, knees bent. Inhale. As you exhale, tilt your pelvis and slowly roll up to a mini or full pelvic tilt.

Benefit: bonds and relaxes both partners, balances the nervous system.

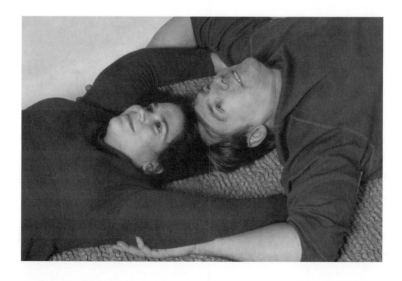

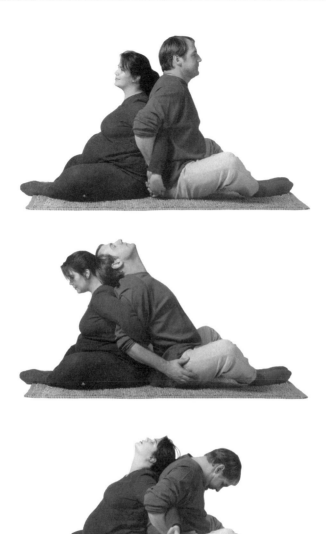

Double Angel—Sit back to back in the butterfly position with your elbows interlaced. Stretch forward while your partner arches back. Then, your partner stretches forward and you arch back.

Benefit: enhances the benefits of the butterfly with the contact of each others' backs.

119

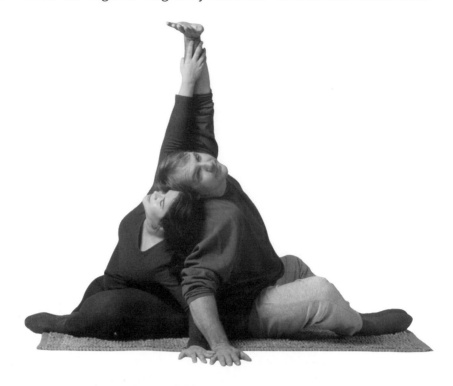

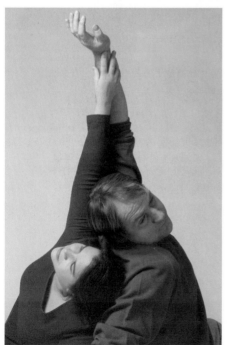

Angel Side Stretch—Sit next to your partner in the butterfly position. Reach over to one side keeping your arm straight and up against your ear, while your other hand remains on the floor and your elbow bends. For a greater stretch hold your partner's hand in the air. Breathe. Switch to the other side.

Benefit: enhances the side stretch, encourages fuller breaths and relaxes the neck muscles.

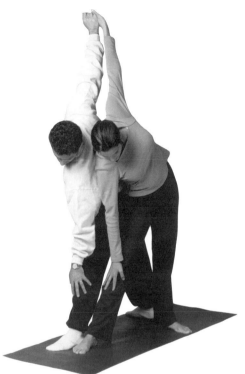

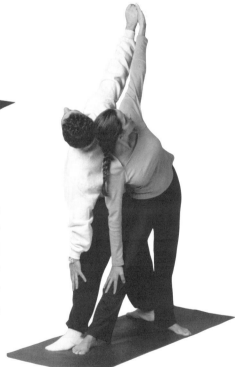

Triangle Lift and Tilt—Stand in the triangle pose with your back to your partner. Your turned-out feet should meet. Both partners should tilt their pelvis and slide their arm down their respective turned out leg. Gaze down and then up.

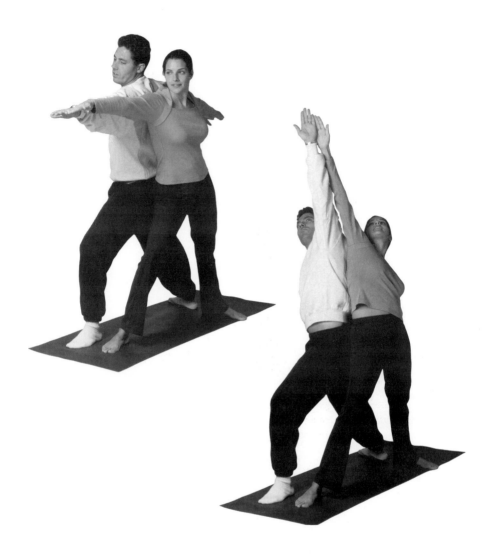

Warrior—Stand back to back. Starting in the triangle pose, bend your turned-out leg, making sure that your knee bends over your foot. Reach your arms out to shoulder height, hands touching your partner's hands. Gaze over your arm on the turned-out side.

Warrior Variation—Reach your arm down to the straight leg. Stretch the other arm up in the air and gaze upward. Breathe. Repeat.

Warrior Side Stretch—From the warrior pose, both partners lean on the thigh of the turned-out leg while stretching your other arm over head. Feel the stretch and breathe.

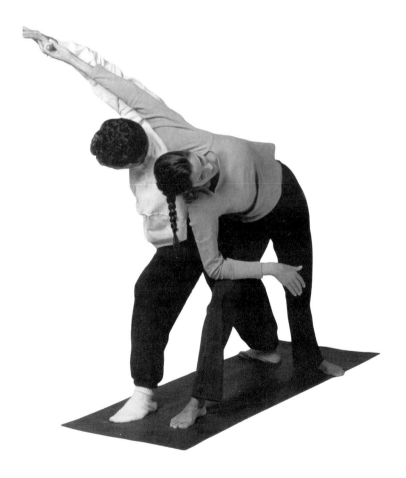

PART VII – PREGNANCY AND POSTNATAL MASSAGE

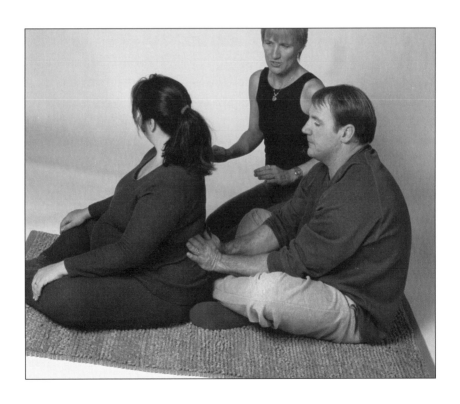

Massage is a wonderful skill to have and anyone can learn to give a short, relaxing massage. On the following pages I present techniques in self-massage, foot massage, pre- and post-natal massage and father massage. Massage is a sensuous, loving way to share and communicate with your partner. It helps you to relax and has many benefits, some of the same that practicing yoga offers. In that way, yoga and massage complement each other.

Couples often have questions about where they can massage and what specific strokes are beneficial during pregnancy. This chapter provides many wonderful massage techniques that can be added onto workouts.

I have worked with many pregnant women and they all say that massage helped so much during their pregnancy. There are several reasons for this. Since your hormone levels are heightened and you are feeling more sensual, it feels particularly great to be massaged.

Massage also relieves pressure on your back due to the weight of the pregnancy and your posture constantly adjusting to the growing baby. In addition, massage helps lymphatic drainage, which has to work harder during pregnancy and postpartum. You have heard of women getting puffy feet and fingers in later pregnancy. Massaging the feet, hands and back helps to limit such swelling. With my second pregnancy, it was hot in July and nothing could relieve my back and my feet like a good massage.

The father of your baby is also under a lot of stress and tension during the pregnancy. He may have concerns about how the pregnancy is going and how having a child will change his life. He deserves a little massage, as much as you have energy for. He will enjoy simply having his shoulders worked on, or having his scalp and face massaged. You want to work as a team throughout the pregnancy.

Receiving your first massage after your baby arrives feels particularly wonderful. My friend Meg, a massage therapist, traveled two hours on the Long Island Railroad to give me a massage after I delivered my first child, Amanda. It felt so great to be able to take that time to go inward and readjust to my body again. Now that the miracle of delivering the baby had occurred, the process of taking care of both my baby and my body had begun.

Postnatal massage offers many of the same benefits as prenatal massage. It increases circulation and enhances the lymphatic system, which reduces swelling. It improves the texture of the skin and reduces or diminishes stretch marks, especially when you use high-quality oils. Massage also releases the tightness that gathers in the shoulders and the middle of the back from holding and nursing your baby. It also helps you bond with your partner sensually after the baby arrives.

Couple massage encourages your partner to breathe fully, even when parts of the body are sensitive to touch. It is important to give each other feedback and sense when your muscles are relaxing. The massage techniques in this chapter can be applied interchangeably to a man or a woman. Remember that both the giver and receiver should be in comfortable positions. You cannot give a good massage if you are uncomfortable.

Aromatherapy Oils

You can practice massage with your clothes on, or you can take your clothes off and complement the treatment with the use of oil or lotion. It is recommended to use a massage oil rich in vitamin E. Since your skin can become dryer during pregnancy, the oil helps to prevent stretch marks and improves skin quality.

Use high quality oils. In early pregnancy I would recommend using grapeseed or an almond oil base, and possibly a small amount of lavender or chamomile essence. High quality oils are uplifting, they improve circulation, increase energy and minimize fatigue. Essential oils for pregnancy can be used in a low dilution because of scent sensitivity. Organic oils are preferred to over-the-counter ones.

I believe tangerine is the best pregnancy oil. It has a pleasant refreshing smell and a harmonizing effect on the body and mind, When combined with jasmine, sambac and neroli, its fragrance is heavenly. Face oils are also very useful when pregnant to smooth your skin and lesson the chance of broken capillaries. Each evening, apply a blend of tangerine, jasmine, chamomile or neroli and grapeseed oil.

Before beginning your massage, check with your doctor, make sure the room is a comfortable temperature, and try to limit interruptions.

COUPLE MASSAGE, PART I

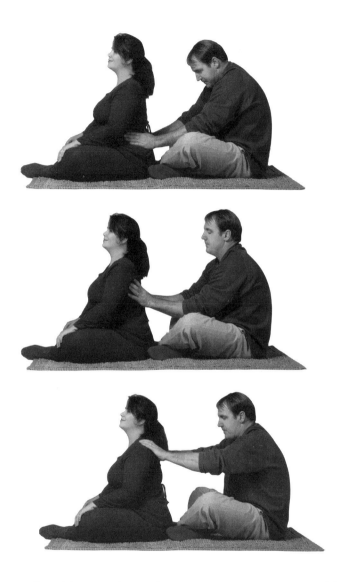

1a. Sit comfortably cross-legged, as your partner warms up his hands by rubbing them together. When ready, your partner gently glides his hands up your back using full palms.

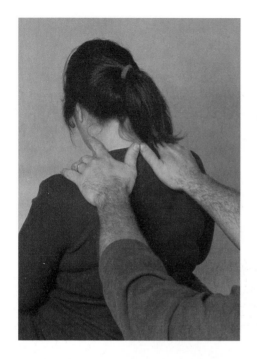

1b. At the top of your shoulders he squeezes twice then glides his hands gently down your back. Repeat three times.

2. Using his thumbs, your partner makes small circles close to your neck. This is followed by three circles in the middle of your trapezius (top of the shoulder), and three circles on the outer trapezius.

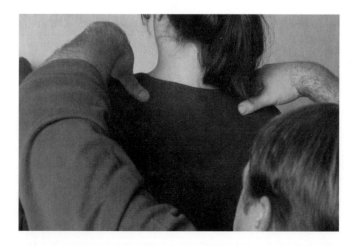

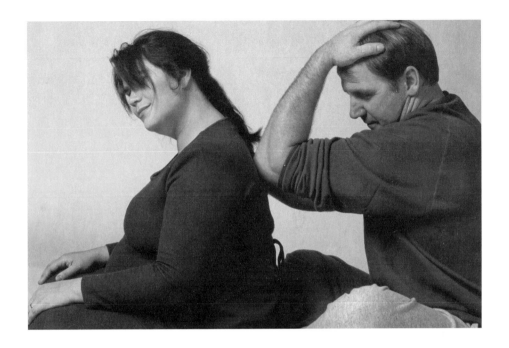

3. Supporting you with one hand, your partner uses his elbow to make small circles
   between your spine and your shoulder
   blade. Take long breaths.

COUPLE MASSAGE, PART II

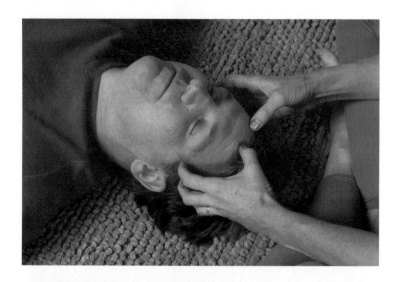

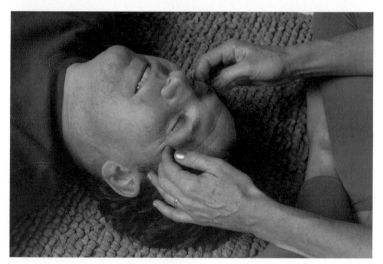

1. With your head, neck and shoulders on the ground, use your index and middle fingers to gently massage your partner's temples in small circular movements.

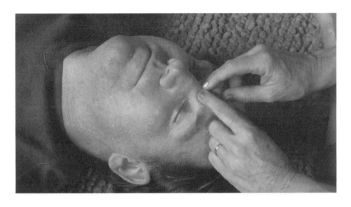

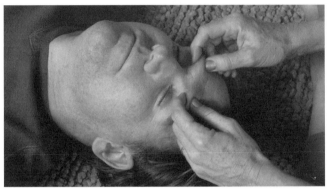

2. Hook your thumbs under the ridge of your partner's eyebrows and squeeze the brow from the inner to the outer three times.

3. From behind your partner, place your hands on the bottom of your partner's neck and use them to stretch and lengthen it.

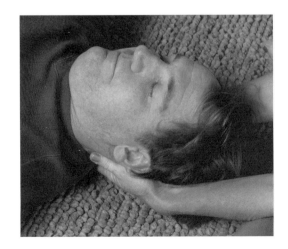

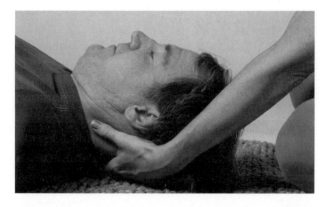

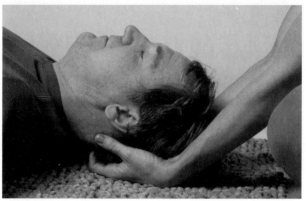

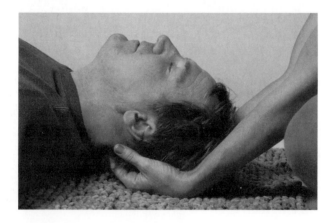

4. Hook your fingertips under the ridge of your partner's head. Hold while you support his neck and tilt his head.

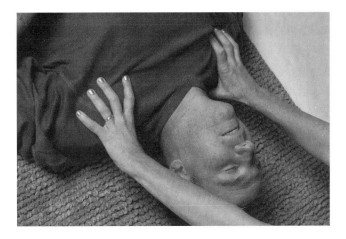

5. Bring your hands to your partner's shoulders and press into the shoulders with your thumbs. Sense where there might be tension and press in that area three to five times.

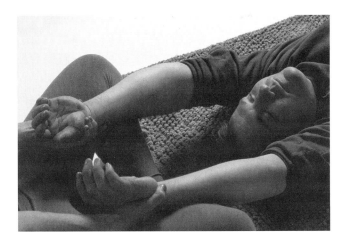

6. Hold your partner's arms and stretch them over his head, reminding him to take deep, full breaths.

COUPLE MASSAGE III

Lie on your side with your top knee bent and a pillow under your head and knee.

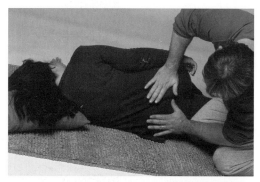

1. Partner places hands flat on your lower back and glides up your back on both side of the vertebra three times.

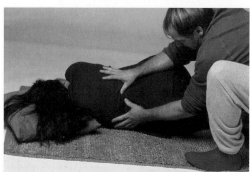

2. With his thumbs, your partner makes small circles up your back near the vertebra, massaging the big muscles that go up the spine three times and then glides down.

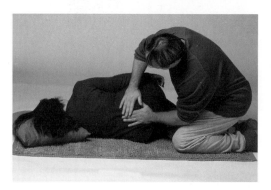

3. Partner makes small circles on the center of the lower back.

4. Partner massages in circular motion with the whole hand around the hips.

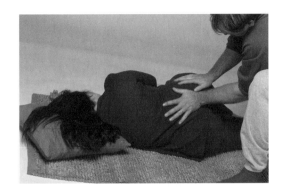

5. Partner places one hand on your shoulder, the other on your hip, and stretches while you exhale.

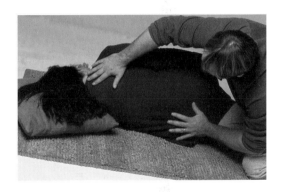

6. Partner uses full palm to "nerve" stroke your back lightly gliding down your back.

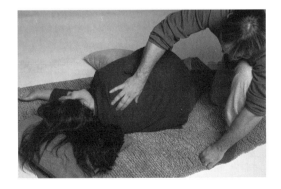

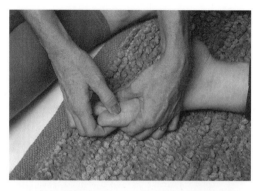

8. Partner continues to work down to your top foot while you remain lying on your side. He kneads the bottom of your foot gently with both hands, from your heel to your toes.

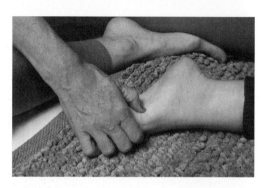

9. Using his thumbs, partner makes small circles up the arch of your foot from the heel to the ball. He presses the bottom of each toe, then stretches each toe.

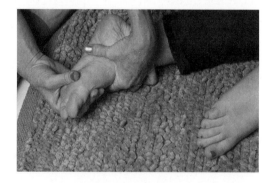

10. Using two hands partner twists your entire foot back and forth three times.

11. Slowly turn to your other side and repeat the massage.

POSTNATAL COUPLE MASSAGE

Lie on your stomach with your head to the side. (Hurray, it is great to be able to lie on your stomach again.)

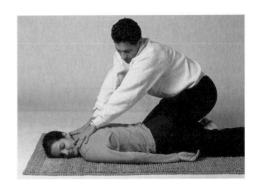

1. Partner uses his full palms to glide up your back, over your shoulders and lightly down again three times.

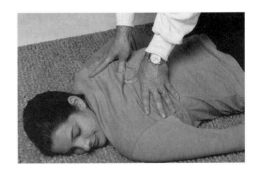

2. Partner uses his thumbs to make small circles close to your spine as he massages up your back.

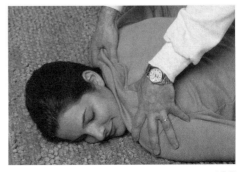

3. Partner should concentrate on tight areas, making small circles there until the muscles loosen up a bit.

139

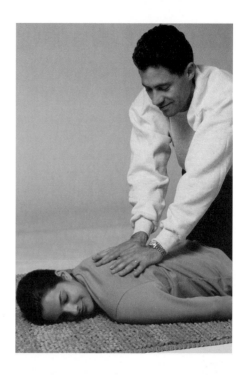

4. Partner rests both palms on the middle of your back while you take three full breaths.

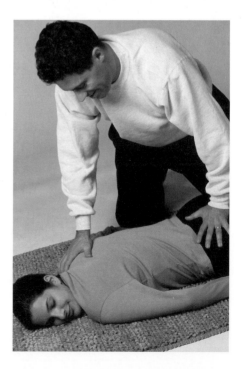

5. Partner places one hand on your left hip, the other on your right hip and stretches to one side while you exhale twice. Then reverse.

Part VIII – Baby Yoga and Massage

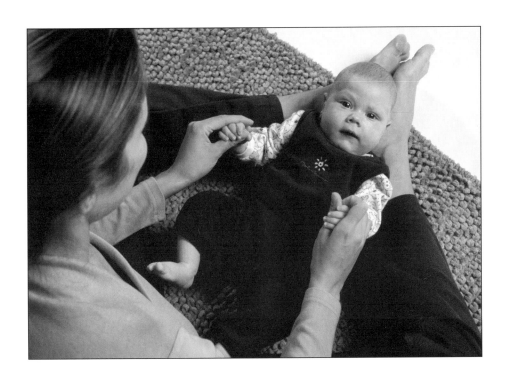

Baby yoga can be a great part of your own workout. I recommend starting some infant yoga when your baby is about six weeks old. Prior to that, you are busy nursing, catching up on sleep and simply sitting and admiring your baby. Remember to check with your pediatrician before you begin.

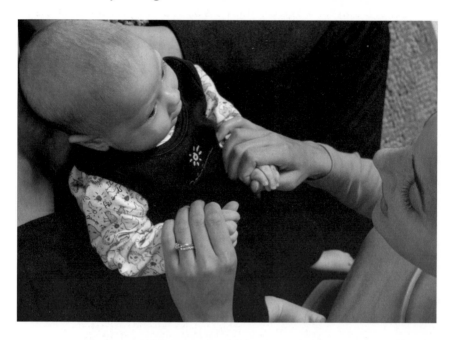

You may begin baby yoga while you nurse your baby, simply by taking full deep breaths and doing some meditation. This is a way to relax and rejuvenate you as well as your baby, helping to increase milk flow. While you nurse, prop one pillow behind you and another one under your baby so you don't round your shoulders and can remain as comfortable and relaxed as possible.

Baby exercises can be a wonderful way to strengthen the bond between you and your baby. The father also should do some of the stretches and massages with the baby so that he may also feel the bond.

Baby yoga provides many benefits for your baby. It gently stimulates the neuromuscular system, and is a great way to help balance the right and left sides. It is fun for the infant to focus his or her eyes on Mommy or Daddy while being stretched. The baby is starting to see in focus and it is important to make eye contact with your baby. In addition, massaging your baby may help relieve colic and gas. Research also indicates premature babies that are held and massaged gain weight more quickly than those that are not.

I believe that massage on infants is as soothing for them as it is for adults. With babies a light touch is necessary and the duration should be short. A little massage goes a long way for a little body. After practicing the massage in the book, observe your baby's response.

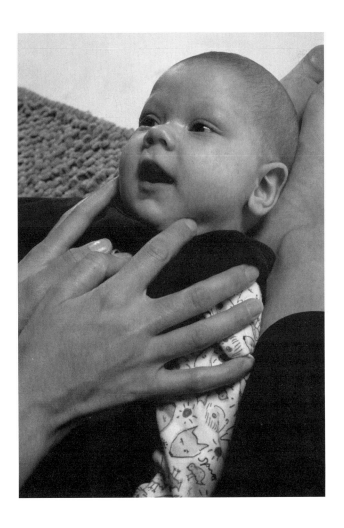

BABY MASSAGE

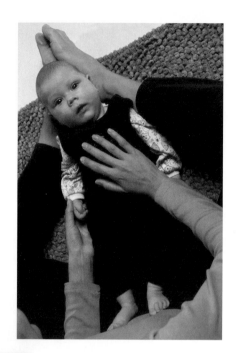

1. Sit in butterfly pose with your baby resting on your feet. Place your hand on the baby's belly and massage clockwise, making three circles.

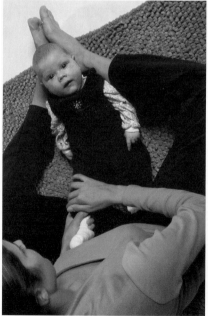

2. Make long strokes up and down each of your baby's legs. Repeat twice.

3. Move down to your baby's feet (around the ankle.) Make small circles on the bottom of the foot and stretch each toe.

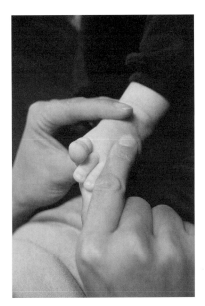

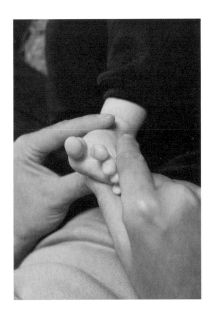

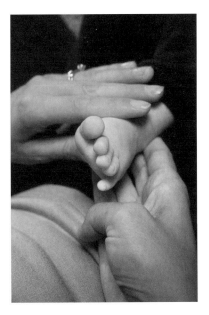

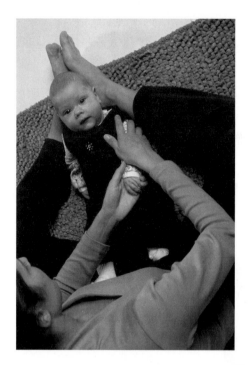

4. Massage up and down each arm.

5. Move to the hands and gently stroke each finger.

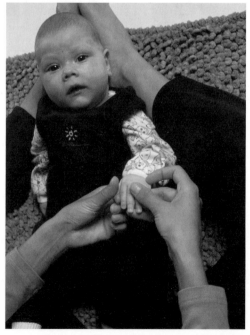

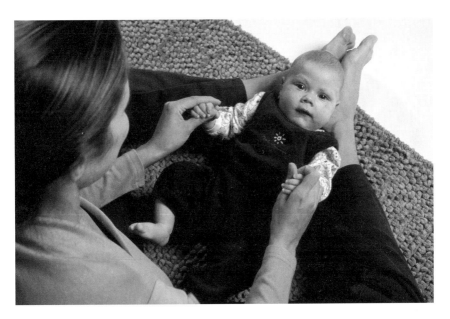

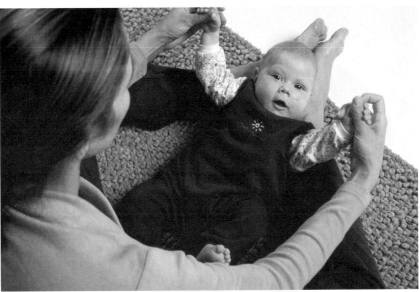

Baby Yoga 1—Sit in the cross-legged or butterfly position. Hold both of your baby's hands, stretching the arms overhead and then bringing them back down. Repeat three times.

Benefit: strengthens arms.

147

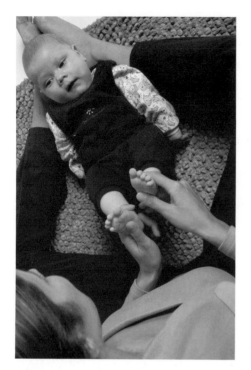
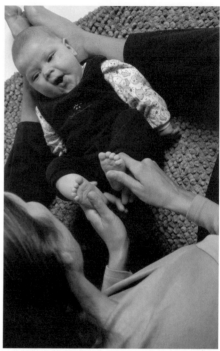

Baby Yoga 2—Then, hold your baby's feet, gently push in towards his or her chest and release. Repeat twice.

Benefit: strengthens hips.

Baby Yoga 3—Cross your baby's opposite hand to foot three times on each side.

Benefit: helps balance left and right sides, relaxes your baby.

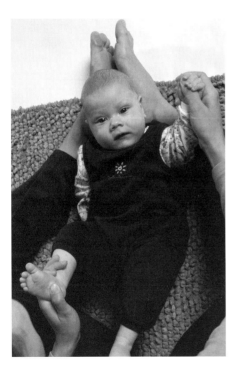
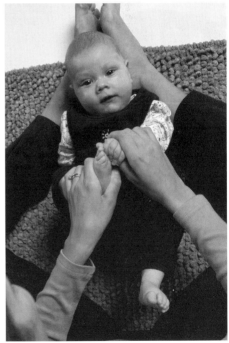

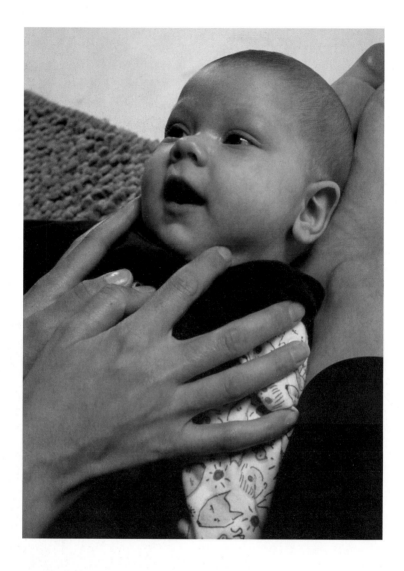

Circle the Face—Using your index finger, lightly circle the outline of your baby's face at least three times.

Benefit: relaxes your baby, makes your baby laugh.

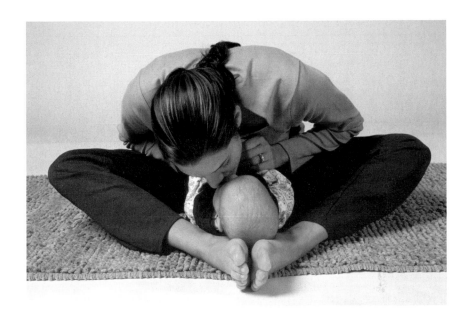

Kiss in Butterfly Pose— While sitting in the butterfly pose, lean forward to kiss your baby. This exercise gives you another reason to stretch a little further and is a great inner thigh stretch.

Benefit: releases tension in your pelvis and lower back. Baby loves this too!

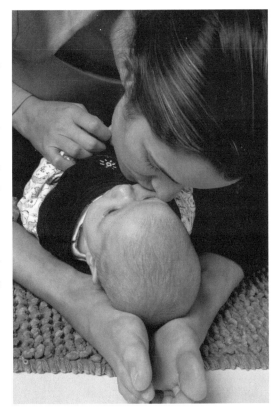

IX – RELAXATION

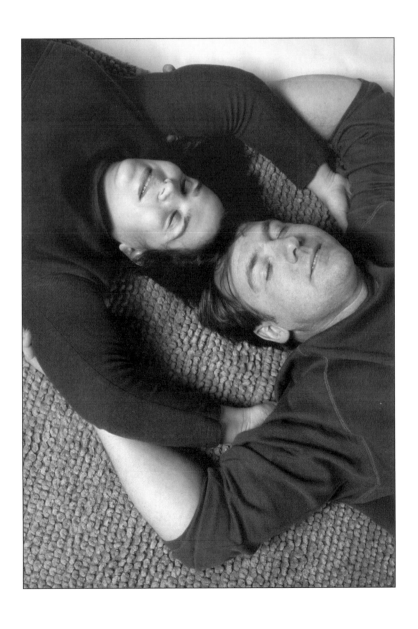

Relaxation and breath work will help rejuvenate your mind and will help you stay more focused when you are in labor. A nice guided relaxation is to lay on your side with one pillow under your head and one under your knee. Close your eyes and imagine drifting off to a Caribbean island. Feel your body sink into the sand, making an impression of your body. Tune into your breathing. Feel the muscles of your back relax. Notice the muscles in between your ribs release. As you inhale your ribcage expands, as you exhale release all tension and worry.

Now tune into your stomach. As you inhale feel that you are breathing down toward your baby. As you exhale imagine what size your baby might be and in what position. You may place your hand on your abdomen. Feel the miracle of your baby growing inside you.

Feel that your baby is in a perfect environment to grow and be born. This is a special time when you and your baby are in the same body. You are taking good care of yourself and feeling positive about the pregnancy. The baby picks up on this and is also in a peaceful state—growing, floating and absorbing all the good nutrients your body is providing.

Now might be a good time to do a set of 30 kegals and then drift into a deep relaxation.

Imagine the sound of the ocean. The inhale and the exhale of your breath are similar to the sound of the waves. As you inhale, your stomach rocks forward and as you exhale it rocks back. You are rocking and soothing your baby into relaxation at the same time.

Labor Relaxation

In early labor when the contractions begin it is good to try to walk around and stretch. Try doing some of the yoga listed in the labor exercise routine. You and your partner will probably sign up for a Lamaze class where you will learn exactly what to expect during the birthing process. I can tell you that it is very important to remain as relaxed as possible. Before the labor progresses, take a walk or a warm shower. Then remember to take long baby breaths whenever possible.

Have your partner and labor assistant massage you, especially in your lower back. Try not to hold your breath. When you are fully dilated, push from your pelvic floor and birth canal muscles, and try to relax your face. Remember that this is the most important time of your life.

As the contractions increase take shorter breaths. I found the "hoot hout" sequence, in which you do the bunny breath while saying "hoot hout," very helpful during contractions, because it gives you the sound to focus on. You release some tension by shouting "hoot hout" at whatever volume you can. I also found it helpful to have a pillow to hug during contractions, as well as some music. During the pushing stage of my labor, I wanted to hear the sound of running water. Perhaps a recording of a waterfall or the ocean would be helpful to play in the background.

PART X — SALUTATIONS

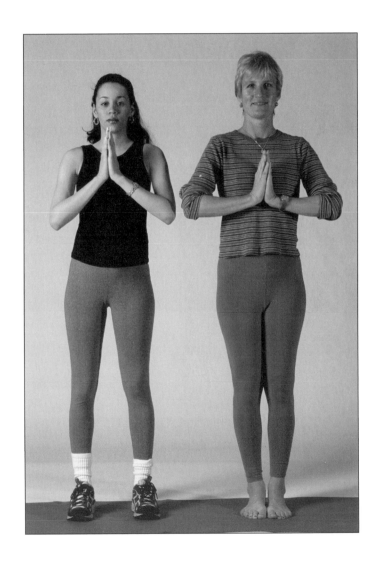

Sun salutations are perfectly balanced yoga progressions. Salutations stretch almost every major muscle group in your body. They incorporate balance, forward bending, backward bending, and neutral exercises. These routines enhance strength and flexibility. Proceed slowly at first, focusing on learning the salutation and the breathing.

PRENATAL SALUTATION # 1

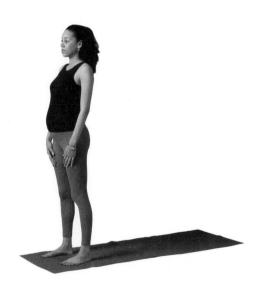

1. Mountain Pose

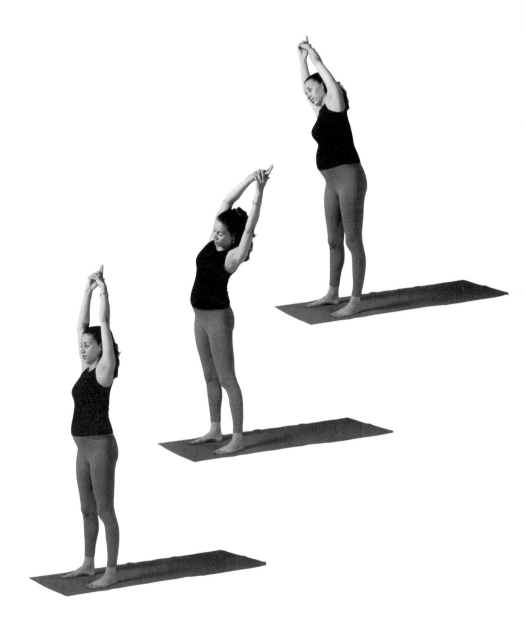

2. Half Moon

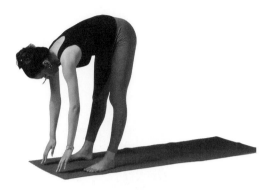

3. Standing Forward Bend

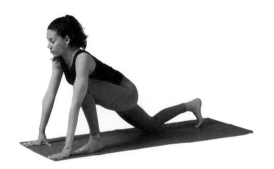

4. Lunge, right leg back

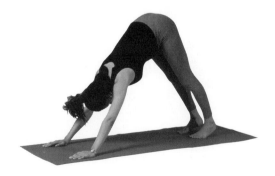

5. Down Dog

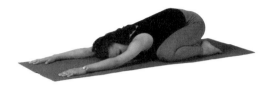

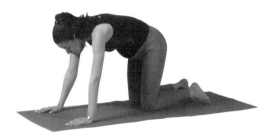

7. Child Pose

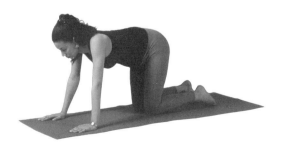

6. Cat Pose

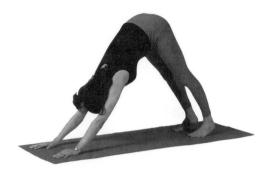

8. Down Dog

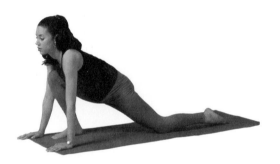

9. Lunge, left leg back

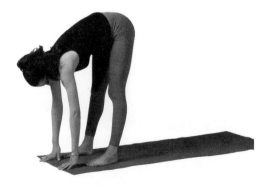

10. Forward Bend

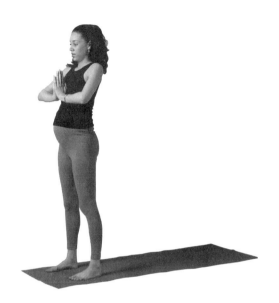

12. Prayer

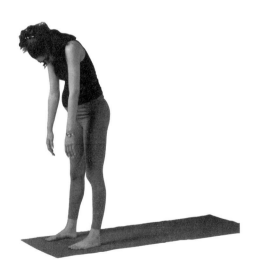

11. Roll Up

PRENATAL SALUTATION #2

1. Prayer
2. Forward Bend
3. Lunge
4. Triangle Lift and Tilt
5. Down Dog
6. Cat Pose
7. Child Pose
8. Lunge
9. Triangle Tilt and Lift
10. Forward Bend
11. Roll Up
12. Mountain Pose

PRENATAL SALUTATION #3

1. Prayer
2. Squat
3. Lunge
4. Warrior
5. Warrior Side Stretch
6. Down Dog
7. Warrior
8. Warrior Side Stretch
9. Lunge
10. Forward Bend
11. Roll Up
12. Prayer

POSTNATAL SALUTATION #1

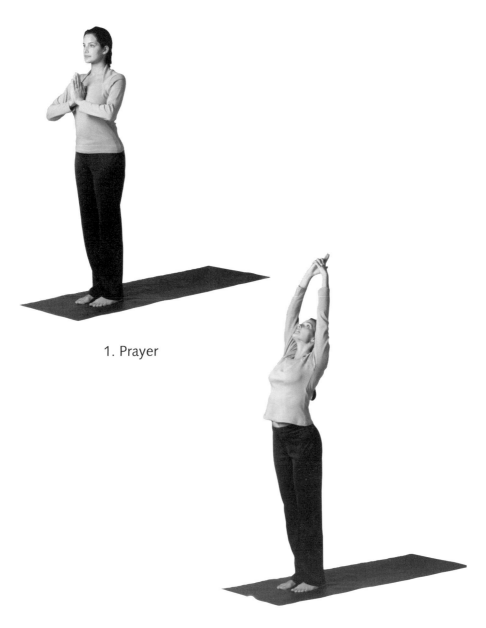

1. Prayer

2. Half Moon Backbend

165

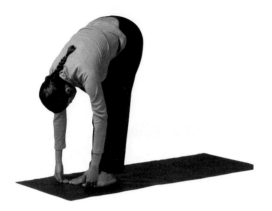

3. Forward Bend

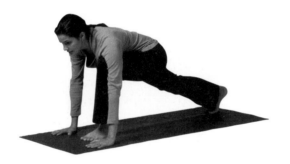

4. Lunge, right leg back

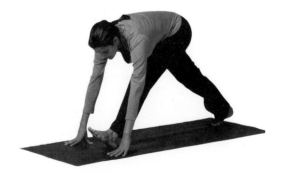

5. Lunge Variation

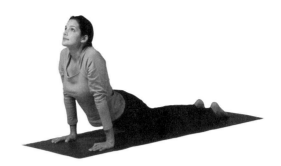

8. Up Dog

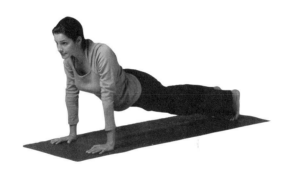

7. Plank

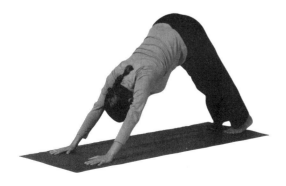

6. Down Dog

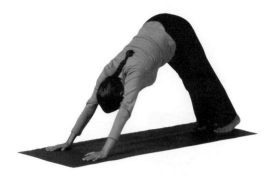

9. Down Dog

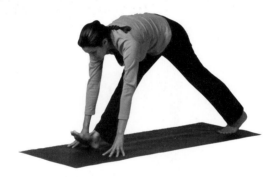

10. Lunge Variation

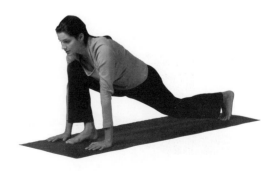

11. Lunge, left leg back

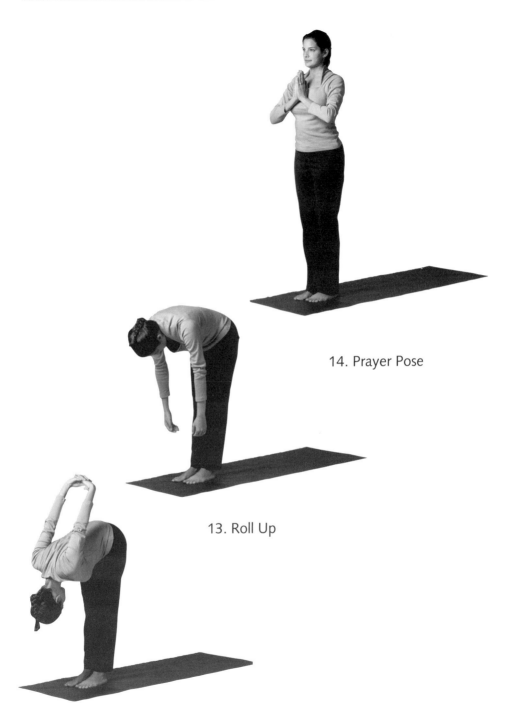

14. Prayer Pose

13. Roll Up

12. Swimmer's Stretch

POSTNATAL SALUTATION #2

1. Prayer
2. Forward Bend
3. Lunge, right leg back
4. Down Dog
5. Warrior, right leg bent
6. Warrior Side Stretch, right leg bent
7. Down Dog
8. Plank
9. Up Dog
10. Warrior, left leg bent
11. Warrior Side Stretch, left leg bent
12. Lunge
13. Roll Up
14. Mountain Pose

PART XI – YOGA ROUTINES

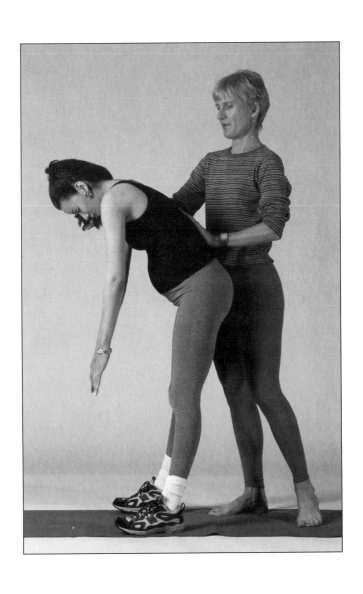

Labor Exercise Routine

Breathing exercises
Child Pose
Pelvic Tilts
Kegels
Double Yoga
Plies
Squats

Three to Six Month 15-Minute Workout

Angel Breath
Chin Rolls
Butterfly
Cross-Legged Spinal Twist
Side Arm to Leg Stretch*
Ankle Rotation*
Side knee lift*
Hip Shaper*
Lying Quad Stretch*
Pelvic Tilt
Cat Pose
Down Dog
Lunge, right leg back
Down Dog
Lunge, left leg back
Standing Forward Bend
Roll Up
Salutation #3
Repeat these exercises on both sides of your body.

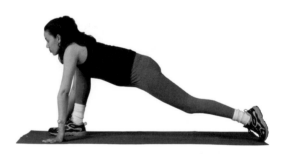

15-Minute Mid-Pregnancy Workout

Prayer
Roll Down
Lunge
Down Dog
Cat Pose
Child Pose
Pelvic Tilts
Kegels
Cross-Legged Position
Seated Side Stretch
Straddle
Half Moon
Plies
Plies Side Stretch
Warrior
Warrior Side Stretch
Chest Expansion
Prayer

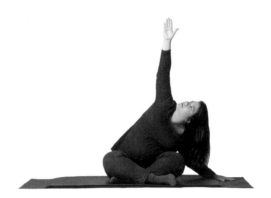

10-Minute Pregnancy Workout (Modified Version)

Half Moon
Triangle*
Triangle Lift and Tilt*
Warrior*
Warrior Side Stretch*
Plies
Squats
Mountain Pose
Tree Pose
Angel Breaths
* Repeat these exercises on both sides of your body.

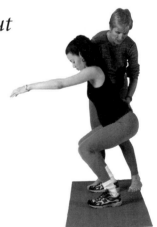

20-Minute Cool Down Three to Six Months

Prayer
Half Moon
Plies
Plie Side Stretch
Pre-Natal Salutation #1
Cross-legged Seated
Kegels
Chest Expansion
Cross-Legged Spinal Twist
Hurdler
Straddle
Straddle Side Stretch
Mini Pelvic Tilts

20-Minute Couple Workout With Massage

Seated Roll Down
Squat
Standing Pelvic Tilt
Suspension Bridge
Hurdler
Double Straddle
Double Bridge
Double Angel
Double Angel Side Stretch
Couple Massage Part I

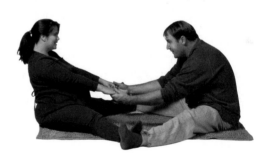

PART XII – NUTRITION

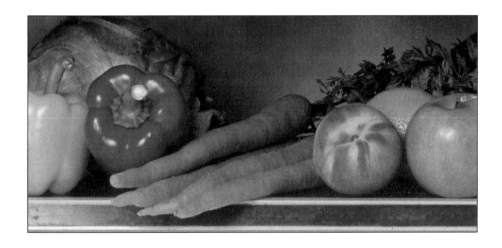

Pregnancy increases your energy needs by 15%. This means that it is necessary to increase calorie consumption by approximately 300 calories daily. One third of these calories is for maternal fat gain, the remainder provides the energy needed for the fetus and increased metabolic activity.

Pregnant women need a slight increase of about 10-15 grams of protein each day. Two additional glasses of milk or one additional serving of protein should provide the extra protein needed.

BASIC DAILY PREGNANCY DIET
Predominant Nutrient

FOOD   SERVINGS

Proteins and Iron ....lean meats, fish, 3-4 oz
                                  Poultry and Lentils, dried beans,
                                  peas, eggs, nuts, 3-7 oz

Protein and Calcium ....milk and cheese, 4 oz

Vitamin C ....citrus fruits and juices, broccoli,
                                  Brussel sprouts, tomatoes and
                                  peppers, 1 or more servings

Vitamin A ....dark green veggies, yellow veggies,
                                  kidney beans, 1 or more servings

Energy and B Vitamins ....whole grains and enriched breads
                                  and cereals, 5 servings

Other Vitamins and Minerals ..all fruits and veggies, 2 or more
                                  servings

Energy Fat and Sugars ....only as needed for energy

VITAMIN & MINERAL REQUIREMENTS

Nutrient	Non-Pregnant	Pregnant	Food Sources
VITAMINS			
Vitamin A	800mg	800mg	dark green or yellow vegetables and fruits, whole milk, eggs and fortified margarine
Vitamin B6	1.6mg	2.2mg	meats, poultry, fish, whole grain cereals, green leafy vegetables, carrots and potatoes
Vitamin B12	2.0mg	2.2mg	meats and poultry
Vitamin C	60mg	70mg	citrus fruits, papaya, strawberries, melon
Vitamin D	5-10mcg	10mcg	fortified milk, sunlight
Folicin	180mcg	400mcg	green leafy vegetables, legumes, liver, orange juice, cantaloupe, whole wheat products
Vitamin E	8mg	10mg	vegetable oil, seeds, nuts, whole grains
Thiamin	1.0mg	1.5mg	pork, beef, nuts, whole grains, wheat germ
Riboflavin	1.2mg	1.6mg	milk, cheese, meats, leafy green vegetables
Niacin	13mg	17mg	fish, meats, peanuts, whole grains
MINERALS			
Calcium	800mg	1200mg	milk, cheese, whole grains, leafy vegetables
Phosphorous	800mg	1200mg	milk, cheese, lean meats
Iron	18mg	30mg	red meat, oysters, cooked spinach, beans
Iodine	150mg	175mg	iodized salt
Magnesium	300mg	450mg	nuts, seafood, whole grains, dried beans, peas

Part XIII – A Final Note

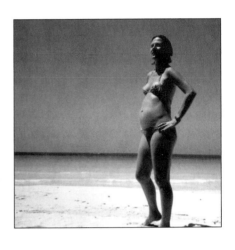

Both of my pregnancies and deliveries were high points in my life. I remember my Aunt telling me that giving birth is like an athletic experience. Someone else told me pregnancy is the time to bond with your child and delivery is the combined effort of you and the baby working together to be born.

As I wrote this book, I reflected on my pregnancies and tried to remember what worked for me. I had such positive pregnancies and relatively easy births, and I think the techniques in this book helped a great deal.

I believe that all the yoga, swimming and walking I did during pregnancy made the births easier. I also feel that staying active and practicing yoga helped me get back into shape and deal with the many emotional challenges of being a mother. Yoga and massage were wonderful techniques for my husband and me to practice together. Once you introduce yoga and massage into your life, you can always call on these techniques.

I hope this book has inspired you to integrate yoga into your life, whether you are trying it for the first time or looking for additional yoga exercises to do during your pregnancy. Enjoy the yoga exercises and massage techniques and of course, enjoy your pregnancy!

Lisa Trivell

Meet the Author

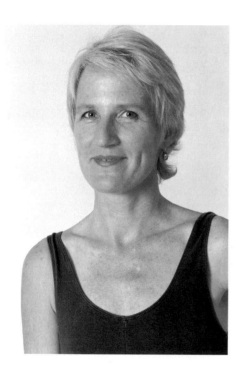

Lisa Trivell is a certified yoga instructor and fitness professional. She is certified to teach yoga, prenatal and postnatal exercise by the International Fitness Professionals Association (IFPA) and the American Aerobics Associations International / International Sports Medicine Association (AAAI / ISMA). Residing in East Hampton, New York, Lisa has two children. She has practiced and taught the techniques in this book for the past ten years and throughout her pregnancies.

BIBLIOGRAPHY

1. Olkin, Sylvia Klein. *Positive Pregnancy Fitness: A Total Approach to a More Comfortable Pregnancy and Easier Birth.* Garden City Park, NY: Avery Publishing Group, 1987.

2. Stillerman, Elaine. *Mother Massage: A Handbook for Relieving the Discomforts of Pregnancy.* New York: Bantam Doubleday Dell Publishing, 1992.

3. The American College of Obstetricians and Gynecologists. *Planning for Pregnancy, Birth and Beyond.* New York: Penguin Books, 1997.

4. Vilim, Reine. (1999, March). *Optimal Pregnancy Fitness.* A manual presented at the AAAI/ISMA Certification Conference, New York, NY.

Congratulations Bridget and Roxanne!

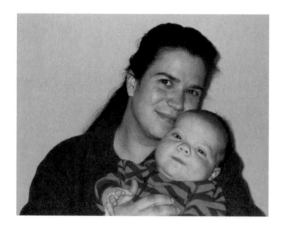

Bridget LeRoy with her baby Bingham Warner Lancelot Johnson, born February 7, 2000.

Roxanne Hughes with her baby Kyree Ronald Meyers, born March 10, 2000.

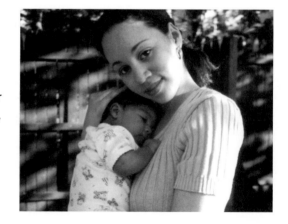

Essence to Essence Aromatherapy

ЭС

Designed by Robin Lyn Shierenbeck.

Offers only organic and wild-crafted essential oils,
Including Chamomile, Lavender, and Juniper!

New Line of Moodbeauty!

Essential oils enhance overall beauty and
well-being and provide an excellent means
of treating discomforts including swelling,
circulation problems, sleeplessness,
stretch marks and nervousness.

Visit her new location:
12 Buckram Road
Locust Valley, New York 11560
Or e-mail Soberbeauty@aol.com

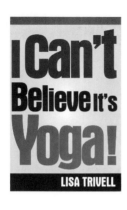

I Can't Believe It's Yoga!

It's Yoga — American Style

Lisa Trivell, Photographed by Peter Field Peck

A popular form of exercise and fitness conditioning, yoga combines stretching and breathing to tone the body, relax the muscles, and relieve tension. The numerous benefits of yoga can easily be added to anyone's daily fitness routine.

For many, though, yoga is seen as being both too difficult and too different to try. *I Can't Believe It's Yoga* addresses this perception problem by presenting a yoga based fitness program which is easy to accomplish.

In *I Can't Believe It's Yoga*, Lisa Trivell, an experienced yoga instructor transforms even the reluctant skeptic into an avid fan. Utilizing the most basic yoga exercises, the results are incredible!

IBSN 1-57826-032-9 / $14.95

Available in bookstores everywhere, order toll free at 1-800-906-1234 or online at getfitnow.com

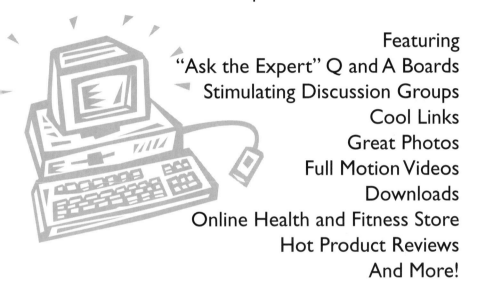

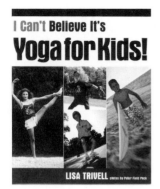